WHAT TO EXPECT

BEFORE, DURING & AFTER A

Hysterectomy

Your Complete Handbook to Prepare
for Surgery, Manage Menopause,
Improve Mindset, and Live Pain-Free

ALLYSON STEWART

What to Expect Before, During & After a Hysterectomy

ISBN #: 979-8-9896392-1-2 | Paperback

Published in the United States of America

Dedication

This book is dedicated to my lovely daughter, who stood beside me throughout my hysterectomy journey. I'm so grateful for you.

Contents

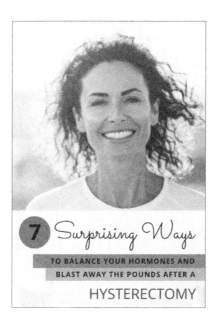

A Special Gift for You!

Included with your purchase of this book is my free guide, *"7 Surprising Ways to Balance Your Hormones and Blast Away the Pounds After a Hysterectomy"*. Use the link or QR code below to grab your copy, and let me know which email address to send it to:

https://www.hysterectomyfitness.com/discover

Introduction

"So you may not always have a comfortable life. And you will not always be able to solve all the world's problems all at once. But don't ever underestimate the impact you can have, because history has shown us that courage can be contagious, and hope can take on a life of its own."

MICHELLE OBAMA

D id you know that one in three women will have a hysterectomy by age 60 and over 500,000 women will undergo a hysterectomy this year? That's just in the U.S. alone. Yet, minimal resources are available to help us cope with this drastic change.

I know because six years ago, my doctor recommended a hysterectomy. I was in debilitating pain from menstrual cramps and suffered from non-stop cycles that had continued for over a year. Large fibroids aggravated the pain, and my life was now at risk.

Hearing the words, "We recommend a hysterectomy," was difficult for me. I was concerned that the side effects would be worse than the agony I was already experiencing.

As an active mom and a career woman, I feared not being at the same fitness level afterward.

To make matters worse, I had read horror stories about women who'd had trouble losing weight after the surgery, and personally, I didn't know if a hysterectomy would fix my gynecological problems.

Additionally, I had seen friends struggle with hot flashes after their procedure, and I didn't want to suffer the same fate and go into menopause right away.

Naturally, I searched for resources — *more like a miracle* — to shrink my fibroids without a hysterectomy and maintain my weight if I proceeded with the surgery.

So, I typed in all my questions online, but what I found wasn't comforting.

There was practically no information for women who wanted to keep the pounds off permanently post-surgery. Instead, the Internet was filled with myths, misconceptions and outdated content at the time.

I delayed my surgery due to a lack of authentic information. But I wish I hadn't.

By the time I finally got to the surgeon, my condition was so bad that he was surprised that I was still functioning. I had severe anemia (6.9 g/dL), was in unbearable pain and felt mentally lost.

After the doctor examined me, he suggested a hysterectomy, but because I didn't want that option, I asked about Accessa (Laparoscopic Radiofrequency Ablation). He mentioned that most insurance companies didn't cover Accessa yet.

Still determined to avoid a hysterectomy, I followed up with questions about a myomectomy. He replied:

> *"A myomectomy could work, but there's no guarantee that the fibroids won't return, and depending on the size and location of your fibroids, we may not be able to remove them all."*

Despite his warning, I decided to proceed with a myomectomy. Big mistake! Within weeks after the procedure, I was back to square one, bleeding heavily and in excruciating pain.

I remember being at work and not being able to walk on my own. A friend had to help me to my car, and I wondered if I should head to the ER right away. Instead, I returned home, praying not to bleed out. Not smart, I know.

It was then that I knew that a hysterectomy was my only option. I contacted the surgeon, and he scheduled an emergency surgery.

I genuinely believe that God saved my life and got me to the doctor in time.

Are you in a similar position? Maybe like me, you're terrified about getting a hysterectomy because you don't know what to expect, but you're also exhausted by the constant battle with pain.

Perhaps you've been told that a hysterectomy is your best bet for survival. Or maybe you're unsure if you're making the right choice by opting for surgery.

You've searched every nook and cranny, but all you've found was conflicting advice and discomforting stories of weight gain, menopause, hormonal imbalance and their effect on women's physical, mental and sexual performance.

And all you want is solid, fact-based advice regarding the entire process. Trust me, you're not alone. I've been there.

I know what it's like to yearn for empathy, support or advice for a hidden health problem; how hard it is to be in a good mood or operate at your best while you're in pain; and how embarrassing it sometimes feels talking about these things or asking for help from others who don't understand how you're feeling.

The Internet has some good resources, but there are more negative voices than positive ones, which can mess with the mind.

Thankfully, it's not all dark and gloomy after a hysterectomy.

I'm proof that you can have a healthy, productive and pain-free life afterward and that you don't necessarily have to be overweight forever, experience never-ending brain fog, lose your libido or any of that awful stuff.

Now, I'm not saying my recovery was easy or that there's a magic pill that got me the results we all want. But there *are* ways.

In this book, I'll share the exact tips, strategies and lifestyle modifications that I use to maintain my fitness and well-being.

This is so you can finally feel at peace with your decision and get the answers you need, even if no one seems to understand what you're going through.

If you are contemplating getting a hysterectomy, or you just got the procedure and are looking for a solution to manage the changes in your body and mind, then Hallelujah! Because you've found it.

This book is a thorough and supportive guide for women like you and me, who are going through this challenge. I've compiled years of research into these chapters to help you feel less alone when facing a hysterectomy.

It was a lonely journey I wouldn't wish on anyone.

Ever since I started to see *significant* and *lasting* results from what I was doing, I made it my mission to share the information with other women like me.

This book is a 360-degree look at the medical, psychological, lifestyle and natural options for navigating gynecological challenges before, during and after a hysterectomy.

You'll find the framework that enables you to enjoy life to the fullest without hysterectomy-related issues limiting you.

I recognize that one size doesn't fit all. As such, I've included *modifiable strategies* you can tweak to suit your needs. But also feel free to follow my plan to a T and reap the benefits, whichever works for you.

Each chapter includes tips to get you back to feeling like yourself again — mentally, physically and emotionally.

The content in this book is a result of six years of study and lots of trial and error. That's more than the time it takes to earn a bachelor's degree.

You'll find information that'll help you manage your health and post-hysterectomy recovery. Like me, you can find joy in your hobbies, work and home life without feeling physically and mentally drained.

Fair warning, though. It can be a challenging journey.

A BIT ABOUT ME

I had a hysterectomy when I was 46. It was an emergency procedure, so I couldn't prepare for it as much as I wanted.

That's something I want to help others with.

If you've scheduled a hysterectomy, there's an entire chapter dedicated to preparing for it, so you can avoid the mistakes I made.

My recovery was a rollercoaster ride. I recall being shocked by how much pain I was in even after the surgery.

My insides felt weird for months. I couldn't exercise or move that quickly (which was super hard because movement is my medicine), and I was gaining weight fast.

I also struggled with unexpected symptoms. For example, I

was surprised that I was still bleeding. I thought that would go away since I no longer had a uterus. In addition, I had a horrible sore throat from the surgery.

I was constipated, which is typical for many women afterward. I needed advice and support with all of this, but it was difficult to find answers from a trustworthy source or to get the information without searching endlessly for it.

Over time, I designed a framework that worked for me. In the process, I learned a lot of other things, too, which *you'll* discover in this book.

I suffered for a long time before I found a tried-and-true system. I don't want you to go through that, so take advantage of my effort and the resources here.

Without further ado, let's get started.

Chapter 1

YOU ARE NOT ALONE

"Don't ever lose hope. Even when life seems bleak and hopeless, know that you are not alone."

NANCY REAGAN

Nearly every woman has heard the word hysterectomy. You may have heard it at the gynecologist's office, around middle-aged women, or from a loved one, colleague or friend.

Since some women talk about it with their eyes squeezed, nose wrinkled and eyebrows furrowed, it's understandable if you associate this term with pain and discomfort.

But do you know what this procedure actually is? Who should get it? Why it's recommended?

Because, spoiler alert: not everyone who gets a hysterectomy has the same issues, nor is it performed the same way on each patient.

If you're considering this procedure, you need to know the facts. And that's precisely what we'll cover in this chapter.

Here's a quick overview:

- What is a hysterectomy? A brief introduction to the types and surgical approaches.

- Who typically gets hysterectomies? Understanding

the influences of age and ethnicity.

- Why hysterectomies are considered an option these days? Helping you decide if it's the correct procedure for you.

- How you may be feeling as you review your options. And my personal experience.

I realize that the topics may sound *science-y*. Still, I'll try not to talk about them like a typical medical professional, b*ut someone who's been through this grueling process myself.* So read it as if you were listening to your friend.

Knowing the facts about the procedure and your options will help you steer clear of misconceptions, so you can make a well-informed decision down the road.

Ready? Let's begin.

WHAT IS A HYSTERECTOMY? A BRIEF INTRODUCTION TO THE TYPES AND SURGICAL APPROACHES.

Hysterectomy is a surgical procedure that removes one or multiple parts of the female reproductive system. This may include the uterus, cervix, ovaries and fallopian tubes.[1]

There are different types of the procedure, but here are the four main categories:

1. TOTAL HYSTERECTOMY:

This type of hysterectomy **removes the uterus and cervix, but not the ovaries.** It's often recommended for women with precancerous cells in their reproductive organs, severe endometriosis, uterine prolapse or other conditions affecting the uterus and cervix.

Unfortunately, it's impossible to get pregnant or menstruate (have periods) after this procedure because the uterus (womb) is removed, but you can still experience pre-menstrual symptoms (PMS).

However, since the ovaries and fallopian tubes are intact, which are essential for fertility, you can still produce eggs. As such, surrogacy remains an option after a total hysterectomy.

2. HYSTERECTOMY WITH SALPINGO-OOPHORECTOMY:

Salpingectomy is the removal of the fallopian tubes, while oophorectomy is the removal of the ovaries. This specific surgery **removes one or both of your ovaries and fallopian tubes.**

If it's a *total hysterectomy*, the uterus and cervix will also be removed. If it's a *radical* hysterectomy with salpingo-oophorectomy, your surgeon will remove the *tissues* surrounding these organs as well.

Salpingo-oophorectomy is the preferred choice for endometrial cancer and trans men and non-binary individuals undergoing gender reassignment surgery.

Since the ovaries and uterus are removed, this type of hysterectomy brings on menopausal symptoms, and you can't get pregnant or produce eggs afterward.

3. SUBTOTAL OR SUPRACERVICAL HYSTERECTOMY:

This hysterectomy removes only the **upper part of the uterus.** It's the ideal choice for non-cancerous conditions like fibroids, endometriosis or heavy menstrual bleeding that's not treatable with other methods.

After the surgery, you'll no longer be able to get pregnant. However, you'll still have menstrual periods since the cervix and part of the uterus are present.

4. RADICAL HYSTERECTOMY:

A radical hysterectomy **removes the uterus, cervix, top portion of the vagina and surrounding tissues.** You may also lose your ovaries and fallopian tubes if it's necessary.

It's the go-to choice for getting rid of cancer. Your fertility options depend on which organs are removed. For example, you can still release eggs if your ovaries remain and are functional.

Now, let's cover the approaches your surgeon can take to complete the various types of hysterectomy.[2] Each has its pros and cons, so it's best to go over them with your surgeon and mutually decide the best approach for you.

1. LAPAROSCOPIC HYSTERECTOMY:

This procedure is sometimes referred to as robotic surgery, although the terms aren't exactly synonymous.

Here, the surgeon removes the uterus through tiny (a few millimeters long) cuts on the lower abdomen. They'll insert a small camera through one of the cuts and, in some cases, two tube-like structures through the other cuts.

The camera helps your surgeon view the inside structures, similar to what they would see if they made a larger, old-school cut. This approach works for removing any of the organs.

The location of the cuts can vary, depending on the surgery type.

A laparoscopic hysterectomy is an outpatient procedure, and you can go home on the same day or within 24 hours.

2. ABDOMINAL HYSTERECTOMY:

In an abdominal hysterectomy, the surgeon makes a six- to eight-inch cut in the abdomen. Again, the cut's location and direction (horizontal or vertical) can differ for different procedures.

This is an in-patient surgery, so you may spend a few days in the hospital. It also has a high recovery time (from two to six weeks).

3. VAGINAL HYSTERECTOMY:

In a vaginal hysterectomy, the surgeon makes a small cut around the vaginal opening to access the organs.

It's less painful compared to the other options, and there are no cuts on your belly. However, a vaginal hysterectomy is not always an option.

WHO HAS HYSTERECTOMIES? UNDERSTANDING THE INFLUENCE OF AGE AND ETHNICITY.

Hysterectomies are most common for women between the ages of 40 - 49.[3]

It's understandable why that's so. Most of the conditions that require any type of hysterectomy occur after the age of 40. But technically, any woman (or non-binary individual) of legal age can consent to the procedure, but it should be medically justified.

It's rare for a surgeon to perform a hysterectomy if you're between 18 - 35 years old unless it's *vital* for your health and no other option will do.

Your ethnicity also plays a significant role in your likelihood of needing or undergoing a hysterectomy.

For example, a U.S. study of women (18 and over), from January 1, 2008 to December 31, 2015, showed that among the 31,385 patients who underwent hysterectomies:[4]

- 49% were White
- 13% were Black or African American
- 21.4% were Hispanic
- 11.5% were Asian
- 5.1% were another race or ethnicity

Here's the data about age from the same study:

- 15.4% were aged 18 to 39 years
- 49.4% were 40 to 49 years old
- 21.9% were between 50 and 59 years old
- 3.1% were older than 59

The study also evaluated the surgical approach for the procedures. They found that 72.9% of hysterectomies were minimally invasive (66% were laparoscopic and 34.0% were vaginal).

Sometimes, **your race also influences the surgical approach your surgeon will recommend.**

A 2022 study evaluated 722 hospitals all over America and found that out of 360,460 patients who underwent a hysterectomy with a minimally invasive approach:[5]

- 56.4% were White
- 14.1% were Black or African American
- 10.6% were Hispanic

- 18.9% were other or unknown race or ethnicity

It showed that black patients were twice as likely than white patients to undergo *open* hysterectomy than minimally invasive surgery.

I'm not a qualified researcher, so I won't jump to conclusions or suggest why these numbers are how they are. I just want to provide all the information you may need to better advocate for yourself.

There's also a difference in the incidence of various diseases among ethnicities. For instance, white women are most likely to be diagnosed with endometriosis.[6] That difference is also a big reason why they are the predominant group undergoing hysterectomies.

However, it's unclear whether biological causes or socioeconomic factors influence the access of different ethnicities to gynecologists and hospitals.

WHY ARE HYSTERECTOMIES CONSIDERED AN OPTION THESE DAYS? HELPING YOU DECIDE IF IT'S THE RIGHT PROCEDURE FOR YOU.

Most women get hysterectomies for the same reasons: cancer, endometriosis, fibroids, cysts, etc. But there are countless other reasons for getting one.[7]

Here are the most common ones.

COMMON REASONS FOR GETTING A HYSTERECTOMY			
Uterine fibroids	Chronic pelvic inflammatory disease	Pre-cancer of the reproductive organs	Uncontrollable heavy menstrual bleeding
Endometriosis	Prolapse of the uterus or vaginal walls	Permanent birth control	Ovarian cysts or tumors
Adenomyosis	Cancer	Gender-conforming surgery	Congenital uterine abnormalities

Do any of these sound familiar? I can relate if they do! Let me briefly explain each one.

UTERINE FIBROIDS

These are non-cancerous (benign) growths of uterine muscles and tissues that can develop at any age. The cause may be unclear. Symptoms of fibroids are heavy bleeding, prolonged periods, pelvic pain and pressure, frequent urination and low back pain.

ENDOMETRIOSIS

The endometrium is a tissue, lining the inmost part of the uterus. Endometriosis is a painful condition where tissues grow in other areas outside the uterus, causing pain or infertility. The main symptom is chronic pelvic pain during periods, but you may also experience lower abdominal pain, pain with sexual intercourse and have difficulty getting pregnant.

ADENOMYOSIS

Adenomyosis happens when the tissue lining the uterus grows into the uterine wall.

You may endure heavy or prolonged menstrual bleeding, severe cramping or sharp pelvic pain during menstruation, chronic pain and discomfort during sex.

CHRONIC PELVIC INFLAMMATORY DISEASE

This is an infection of any organ of the female reproductive system. It can be a sexually transmitted infection. Symptoms include pain in the lower abdomen and pelvis, unusual or heavy vaginal discharge with a foul odor, pain and/or bleeding during sex, fever and a burning sensation when urinating.

PROLAPSE OF THE UTERUS OR VAGINAL WALLS

The muscles and tissues surrounding the uterus or vagina become weak or damaged, causing them to sink into the exterior parts of the vagina.

You may feel heaviness or pressure in the pelvis, tissue protruding from the vagina and have difficulty urinating.

CANCER

Cancer is when your cells grow uncontrollably and spread

to other parts of the body, forming clusters or tumors. It can happen in any organ of the reproductive system.

PRE-CANCER OF THE REPRODUCTIVE ORGANS

This term refers to the abnormal growth of cells that may develop into cancer if they're untreated.

UNCONTROLLABLE HEAVY MENSTRUAL BLEEDING

Also known as menorrhagia, the criterion is vague. Gynecologists describe "heavy bleeding" as bleeding for longer than a week, soaking one or more sanitary pads or tampons every hour for several hours nonstop, passing blood clots that are larger than a quarter, or having to change pads or tampons during the night.

PERMANENT BIRTH CONTROL

Removing the uterus stops you from getting pregnant, so hysterectomies are sometimes used as birth control.

OVARIAN CYSTS OR TUMORS

Cysts are fluid-filled sacs that form within or on the ovaries. They can be cancerous or non-cancerous. You may experience pain, bloating and changes in bowel or bladder habits.

GENDER-CONFORMING SURGERY

Hysterectomies help trans men and non-binary individuals match their self-identified gender.

CONGENITAL UTERINE ABNORMALITIES

Congenital uterine abnormalities are rare, but happen when the uterus develops differently. You may not have any symptoms or know they are there until puberty. They can produce painful cramping, pain during intercourse and repeat miscarriages or premature births.

This list is not exhaustive. You can get a hysterectomy for other reasons as well. Conversely, you can have any of these conditions (or multiple conditions) and not need a hysterectomy.

Hysterectomy should be the last option, and doctors often explore other treatments before recommending it.

Someone you know may have the same gynecological problems as you or even share a diagnosis. Still, your treatment options may vary because of how your body reacts to medication compared to that person.

It took me a while to really understand and accept that.

When I was investigating treatment options to manage my symptoms, I tried natural remedies, switching to healthier meals and exercising regularly. However, I wasn't getting the same results as other women I read about.

That led me to constantly question what I was doing, giving rise to negative emotions. Little did I know that my fibroids had gotten so out of hand that I needed medical attention to eliminate them.

Having conversations with my gynecologist and fellow women helped me overcome the — for the lack of a better word — *resentment* I felt for having such luck.

It's normal to feel like you drew the short stick when it comes to these things. But try not to compare yourself with others as much as you can.

And don't think your doctor is wrong if they recommend a hysterectomy for a condition that's not on this list, which others manage non-surgically. Every woman's body is unique. And post-hysterectomy life can be good, too. I am proof of that.

HOW YOU MAY BE FEELING AS YOU CONSIDER YOUR OPTIONS, BASED ON MY PERSONAL EXPERIENCE

Anxiety, confusion, mental exhaustion, fear of the outcome, stress about the hysterectomy not working out, pain, menopausal concerns, restlessness, loneliness. These are just a handful of the feelings you may experience. I know because I experienced them, too.

You may also have some positive emotions, such as relief that the pain will finally be over; that you'll get your energy back and feel more like yourself again. *But feelings are tricky and can sneak up on you without warning.*

To prepare for these unexpected emotions, be proactive.

Create a system for dealing with both positive and negative thoughts. Find a village of women you can rely on. Educate your family, friends and colleagues on ways to support you through this journey.

Check with your gynecologist to see if they can connect you with other women who have had a hysterectomy and now volunteer to support those weighing their options. If you have that choice, take advantage of it.

I remember being a complete wreck when other alternatives failed and a hysterectomy was my only option.

- I was concerned about weight gain, body shape, mood imbalances and physical activity levels.

- I was confused about the negative information out there, which made me question my decision, and I felt doomed no matter what.

- I was secretly envious of other women who seemed to have normal periods and didn't have to take time off because of menstrual problems. At the same time, I was afraid that a hysterectomy would not fix my pain and health issues.

- I also felt alone — like a lot of my family and friends couldn't relate because they hadn't gone through it.

- But above all, I was thinking about going into menopause and ways to combat that.

Long story short, my mind was like a maze, anticipating worst-case scenarios at every turn. It was overwhelming, and

I was emotionally and mentally drained!

But as with most things, many of my fears didn't come to fruition. I realized much later that most of my anxiety was based on misconceptions, and I feel a bit silly now that I know better.

Misconceptions about something as serious as a hysterectomy should not be taken lightly. Hence, I've dedicated the next chapter to setting the record straight on some of the most common misconceptions about this surgery. Let's see if you, too, believe in any of them.

I understand that this topic may trigger painful memories, so take a break if it gets to be too much. Refresh your mind whenever you need to. Soak in some sun. Take a nice walk. Sip your iced coffee, then get back to this book when you're ready. I'll be here.

Chapter 2

MYTHS AND MISCONCEPTIONS

"All truth passes through three stages. First, it is ridiculed. Second, it is violently opposed. Third, it is accepted as being self-evident."

ARTHUR SCHOPENHAUER

B y now, you must know that I had a lot of misguided ideas about hysterectomy and its long-term effects. That's because I, unfortunately, came across horror stories and outdated information about other women's experiences before I had the procedure.

Don't get me wrong. This surgery is an enormous undertaking and can have unexpected risks, so some of the horror stories are *justified*.

Also, some concerns are based on legitimate issues, such as known malpractice by unscrupulous surgeons. For example, *some* doctors have recommended unnecessary hysterectomies to women to prevent uterine cancer.

Few other surgeons have used hysterectomies as a permanent form of birth control or involuntary sterilization without the patient's consent. As such, it's understandable why there's so much worry and hesitation around this subject.

Another primary reason for the confusion is that the procedure treats *multiple* conditions, so you may have a different presentation.

The recovery also looks different based on the surgical approach and type of hysterectomy.

Everyone errs on the side of caution when it comes to important health matters. I did the same. But as I've mentioned before, that almost cost me my life because I waited too long and got to the hospital in the *nick of time.*

As it turns out, I'm not the only one who's suffered from the lack of authentic and reliable guidelines for hysterectomy patients. It regularly happens to countless women around the world.

In fact, a 2015 study performed on women on their experiences and feelings before and after their hysterectomy found a gap in this area. They reported:

> *"A need for increased education and empowerment in the hysterectomy decision-making process, along with expanding information given for postoperative expectations."*[8]

> *BOSSICK ET AL., 2018*

It's time to set the record straight about some common hysterectomy myths.

MYTH 1: YOU'LL ALWAYS GO INTO MENOPAUSE IMMEDIATELY AFTER A HYSTERECTOMY.

Contrary to popular belief, this isn't always true. Sadly, I was guilty of believing it, too.

TRUTH #1: YOU'LL GO INTO MENOPAUSE ONLY IF YOUR OVARIES ARE REMOVED.

It's your ovaries, not your uterus, that provide estrogen. Since the ovaries are *sometimes* removed during a hysterectomy, many people understandably, but mistakenly, think that it's always part of the procedure. Hence the myth that everyone becomes menopausal after the procedure.

Feel free to go back to Chapter 1 to review the types of hysterectomies and see which ones remove the ovaries.

Women *under 50* typically keep their ovaries during surgery unless the underlying issue stems from the ovary itself. An example of this is severe endometriosis.

You have the right to discuss your options with your doctor and choose to keep your ovaries if they're healthy. That way, you won't go into menopause immediately.

TRUTH #2: YOU ARE TWICE AS LIKELY TO EXPERIENCE OVARIAN FAILURE AND GO INTO PRE-MENOPAUSE MUCH EARLIER AFTER THIS PROCEDURE.

Unfortunately, a hysterectomy has some unpleasant side effects. For example, you are twice as likely to experience ovarian failure and go into pre-menopause sooner than you would have without the surgery.[9]

Additionally, since both the ovaries and uterus play a role in hormone maintenance and regulation, you'll likely experience hormonal imbalances even if you keep your ovaries but remove the uterus or part of it.

Hormonal imbalance is one of the main challenges of post-hysterectomy life, and we'll discuss it in detail in a later chapter.

This fear of early menopause and being menopausal immediately after a hysterectomy makes some women feel like less of a woman.

I've lost count of women who believe they'll be *incomplete, less feminine or defective* after the procedure.

Every time I read something like that or hear a woman say those words, I want to give her the biggest hug and tell her that her femininity is a cluster of so many things, not just her organs. Women are remarkably strong and beautiful. No surgery can take that away. Always remember that.

MYTH 2: A HYSTERECTOMY ALWAYS AFFECTS YOUR LIBIDO AND ORGASM.

This myth is loosely linked to hormonal imbalance and menopausal fears. Let's find out what science says, shall we?

TRUTH: CHANGES IN LIBIDO AND ORGASM DEPEND ON THE TYPE OF HYSTERECTOMY AND PSYCHOLOGICAL FACTORS.

Libido, sexual functioning and the ability to reach orgasm differ from person to person. Additionally, your emotional, mental and physical state after the surgery influences your sex drive, vaginal lubrication and experience.

Changes in libido and orgasm after a hysterectomy depend on a few key factors, such as:

- **Nerve endings** that are removed during the procedure

- **Hormone imbalance** due to the removal of the uterus and/or ovaries

- **Menopause** or perimenopause

- **Mental health** and emotional state

The nerves around the cervix (the connection between the uterus and vagina) are essential for pleasure, sex drive and orgasm. If the entire uterus is removed with or without a significant part of the vagina, there's a chance that these nerves will be cut, decreasing your libido.[10,11]

On the other hand, if the nerves are intact but the ovaries and/or uterus are removed, the changes in hormone regulation can cause vaginal dryness and impact your sex drive.[12]

You'll be happy to know that you probably won't feel much difference in your vaginal sensations during sex compared to before, nor will it feel too odd for your partner — even if an extensive section of the vaginal canal is removed.

Surgeons consider these factors and sew the top of the vagina (vaginal cuff) during a total or radical hysterectomy, so you can still have a healthy sex life afterward.

You also have to account for the fact that women are typically close to menopause when they get a hysterectomy. Being in the pre-menopausal state may decrease sex drive, reduce vaginal lubrication and increase difficulty with orgasm.

The bottom line is that *many* women still enjoy sex and orgasm after a hysterectomy. Some women say their sex lives improved afterward because sex is no longer painful. Others don't desire sex as much after the procedure or can't orgasm.

The more extensive the surgery, the higher the chance of it negatively impacting your libido, sex and orgasm.

The good news is that there are solutions for improving sexual desire and performance.

For example, you can ask your gynecologist for vaginal lubrication creams or medications to regulate your hormones. However, these aren't suitable for everyone, *especially* if the cream contains estrogen or if your hysterectomy was due to cancer.

Some lubricants can increase your chance of heart attack, cancer, stroke, liver problems, blood clots, yeast infection and skin irritation, so always check with your doctor before using them.

Nevertheless, don't let this myth keep you from moving forward with surgery if it fixes a larger issue.

MYTH 3: THE ONLY OPTION TO TREAT GYNECOLOGICAL PROBLEMS IS A HYSTERECTOMY.

Nope. It's the exact opposite.

TRUTH: HYSTERECTOMY IS THE LAST OPTION FOR ISSUES WITH THE FEMALE REPRODUCTIVE SYSTEM.

Hysterectomy is a major surgery, even with a laparoscopic or minimally invasive approach. Because it can influence hormonal regulation, periods, childbearing options and mental health, careful planning and decision-making are essential. It may take months or even years to weigh all your options.

Your gynecologist should aim to get you healthy as safely and painlessly as possible, even if that means non-surgical alternatives.

In some cases, a hysterectomy may be inevitable. For example, if you have uterine cancer or suffer from abnormal bleeding, immediate treatment may be required. The latter was true for me. Other possibilities your doctor may explore include:

Medication

Your doctor can prescribe birth control pills or other types of hormonal birth control to manage uterine fibroids and other conditions non-surgically. In addition, anti-hormonal agents or hormone modulators (such as selective progesterone receptor modulators) can ease the symptoms of your fibroids and decrease their growth.[13]

Endometrial Ablation

This surgery uses electric currents, microwave energy and freezing to destroy the inner lining of your uterus. I know it sounds extreme, but it can get rid of tiny uterine fibroids and treat uterus problems.

On the other hand, it decreases your chances of getting pregnant and increases complications during pregnancy.

Myomectomy/Myolysis

Myomectomy removes uterine fibroids without removing the uterus, an option for women who may want to get pregnant. Your surgeon inserts a small instrument through the vagina and cervix into the uterus to cut tissue using electricity or manually cutting the fibroid with a blade.

Myolysis is another procedure that uses heat or cold energy to destroy fibroids.

Uterine Artery (Fibroid) Embolization (UAE)

UAE is a relatively minor surgery that treats conditions in and around the uterus, such as benign overgrowths and fibroids. It blocks the artery from supplying blood to the uterus and shrinks fibroids by starving them, but the fibroids may eventually return. Because UAE impacts the uterus, it can potentially upset your hormones.

Non-Hormonal Therapy

All medications and treatments that don't involve injecting you with hormones fall under the umbrella of non-hormonal therapy.

For example, vaginal moisturizers or FemiLift Vaginal Laser Therapy can improve vaginal atrophy in women who cannot take estrogen. Acupuncture, lifestyle changes, diet and herbal supplements are also part of these treatments.

Their effectiveness varies from person to person.

Uterosacral Ligament Hysteropexy

This procedure places a mesh-type structure inside your pelvic and uterus areas to resolve uterovaginal prolapse. Kegel exercises and pelvic floor physical therapy can further reduce prolapse post-surgery.

If you're contemplating a hysterectomy, list all your options and put a hysterectomy at the *bottom*.

Only make a decision after you've exhausted all the possibilities and discussed your list with your doctor.

MYTH 4: THERE WILL BE A BIG EMPTY SPACE WHERE MY UTERUS IS.

I felt this way too, but that's not entirely true. Our bodies are incredibly adjustable *and don't get enough credit.*

TRUTH: THE BOWEL AND OTHER ORGANS SHIFT INTO THAT SPACE.

The uterus expands to hold a baby when you're pregnant. The other organs make room to give the baby all the space it needs.

Although a hysterectomy is opposite, a similar thing happens. Your intestines move around and fill the space where your uterus was, but it takes time for the organs to adjust.[14]

I didn't know that before my surgery. That's why I was shocked by the pain I experienced during the ride back home. All my insides felt like they were shaking, and I could feel every bit of it.

Regrettably, I was unprepared and didn't have a pillow to hold onto. I encourage you to bring one along. You'll be glad you did.

Although this shuffling fixes the empty space issue over time, it can give rise to a few other problems.

Your intestines may move too low into your pelvic floor, and there's a possibility of vaginal prolapse. Your surgeon will apply stitches to reduce this risk. Kegel exercises can also strengthen the pelvic floor muscles.

MYTH 5: IF I HAVE A HYSTERECTOMY, I MUST TAKE 6 WEEKS OFF TO RECOVER.

Because there are various types of hysterectomies and surgical approaches, their recovery time also differs. I've listed the typical recovery periods below, but don't beat yourself up if yours takes longer.

TRUTH: RECOVERY TIME DEPENDS ON THE TYPE OF HYSTERECTOMY – WITH MINIMALLY INVASIVE SURGERY HAVING THE QUICKEST RECOVERY. IT MAY TAKE YOU LONGER OR SHORTER TO HEAL, DEPENDING ON WHY YOU HAD THE PROCEDURE IN THE FIRST PLACE.

A total hysterectomy with an abdominal approach is a major procedure. You may need to remain in the hospital for a few days after the procedure.

Comparatively, a laparoscopic vaginal hysterectomy, while also being a major surgery, is done with less tearing and cuts, and you can leave the hospital on the same day.

The more extensive the procedure, the longer the recovery.

Here are the general guidelines:[15]

- Abdominal hysterectomy: 4-6 weeks
- Vaginal hysterectomy: 3-4 weeks
- Laparoscopically-assisted hysterectomy: 2-3 weeks

Personally, I had a laparoscopic hysterectomy and took 3 weeks off. I then worked remotely for 2 additional weeks before returning on-site.

I was still in pain during the remaining weeks and was grateful for the opportunity to stay home, rather than rush back into the office.

Extensive surgeries need more recovery time because more structures are healing. For instance, open abdominal surgeries require general anesthesia and extensive cuts. As a result, you may wake up with a sore throat. Your surgeon may also insert a tube at the incision site to drain excess fluids.

You can use these recommendations to calculate your leave time while you heal.

You may need more or less, depending on your health condition before the surgery, complications during the procedure, lifestyle requirements, and your support needs. The support may be emotional, physical, mental, financial, professional or all of the above. As you gauge your recovery, remember that many factors influence the time, and these vary for everyone.

My goal for elaborating on these misconceptions isn't to paint hysterectomies in a positive light, but to ensure you have the facts before you move forward with a decision.

Here's a quick recap of what we've covered so far:

- **Truth:** You'll go into menopause immediately only if your ovaries are removed.

- **Truth:** Changes in libido and orgasm depend on the type of hysterectomy and psychological factors.

- **Truth:** Hysterectomy is the last option for issues with the female reproductive system.

- **Truth:** The bowel and other organs shift into place once the uterus is removed.

- **Truth:** Your recovery time depends on the type of hysterectomy, with minimally invasive surgery having the quickest recovery. It may take you longer or shorter to heal, depending on why you had surgery.

So, how do you make such an important decision that can have a domino effect with lasting impact? We'll review that next.

Chapter 3

FACING THE DECISION: PROS, CONS & POSSIBLE COMPLICATIONS

"We are drowning in information, while starving for wisdom. The world henceforth will be run by synthesizers, people able to put together the right information at the right time, think critically about it, and make important choices wisely."

EDWARD O. WILSON

G etting a hysterectomy is a big decision with no return policy. Doubt creeps in, and it's easy to feel indecisive. But since no one else can make the decision for you, reviewing the pros, cons and possible complications can help you narrow down your choices.

A hysterectomy wasn't my first choice.

I tried medication, natural remedies, exercise, nutrition and a myomectomy before my procedure. The only reason I decided to go with the hysterectomy was because it could save my life.

Even though I knew it was the right surgery for me, the decision was still tough. I was terrified of making the wrong move. Thankfully, I found solace in God. Additionally, I took steps to calm my nerves, which I'll discuss here.

If you're wrestling with your decision, too, apply the tips from this chapter. They can make a world of difference and give you confidence, regardless of your election.

DON'T BE AFRAID TO ASK QUESTIONS

No question is too silly when the stakes are high, so don't feel embarrassed to ask your gynecologist any questions that are troubling you.

Even if you've already asked a hundred questions, knowing what to expect is better than not knowing, then kicking yourself later because you could have tried something else.

If your doctor forces you to rush to a decision, dismisses your questions, or bullies you in any way, take that as a sign to seek a second opinion.

In fact, you should get a second medical opinion even if all your questions are answered. There's no harm in that. It's a common healthcare practice.

Here are some basic questions you can ask:

- Will the procedure only treat the symptoms, or will it permanently fix the underlying issue?

- If I don't have the surgery, what will happen?

- What other treatment options do I have?

- If I don't get a hysterectomy, will my symptoms go away naturally with menopause?

- Can the problem return after the procedure?

- If I want a child in the future, can I preserve my eggs via a surrogate, for example?

- What type of hysterectomy would you recommend? What are its risks, benefits and side effects?

- Should I expect any complications during and after the procedure? Can you describe them and share their statistics?

- How much will the procedure cost?

- Who will perform the surgery and anesthesia, and what are their qualifications?

- Which structures will you remove and why?

- How and when will I get the test results?

- Have you performed this specific surgery before? What's your success rate?

- Can you connect me to a support group for women who've had a hysterectomy?

- Will I need to follow up after the surgery? How frequently and when?

Feel free to modify these questions and add your own.

HOW TO MAKE BIG DECISIONS CONFIDENTLY

Making big decisions when there's not enough information is tough. It's even more challenging when there's a fast-approaching deadline and you're in a lot of pain or not feeling your best.

Top leadership experts have a process they follow when they're faced with life-changing decisions.

I've found their tips so beneficial that I now apply them whenever I'm at a crossroads. I hope you'll find them helpful, too. Let's review them together.

WHAT IS THE ROOT PROBLEM?

Identify *why* you're considering a hysterectomy. I'm not talking about your symptoms, but the actual problem you're seeking a solution for.

Determine whether the problem is big enough that it requires major surgery or if there are other options you can try to fix the root issue.

UNDERSTAND YOUR OPTIONS

Identify your goals. Your options will change based on what you hope to achieve through the surgery.

For instance, a total hysterectomy may be an option if you don't want to get pregnant. In contrast, it might not if you want to keep your uterus.

List your goals. Share them with your gynecologist and ask what your choices are based on your preference.

Research each alternative to learn their pros and cons, then weigh your options to decide what's best. I like to list each procedure in a separate column on a page so they're side by side. I then jot down the benefits and drawbacks for each one.

This activity will give you a clear picture of what you'll gain or lose without a hysterectomy and whether an option is important enough to consider.

WHAT ELSE CAN BE DONE OR TRIED?

Create a checklist of all treatment possibilities and confirm that you've explored them.

Speak with your gynecologist and other women who have a similar condition to see if your list should include anything new.

Add those too if you're a suitable candidate.

HYSTERECTOMY ALTERNATIVES (N.D.)		
Alternative treatments	**Condition(s) it treats**	**Additional information**
Dilation and curettage (D&C)	Abnormal bleeding	This treatment involves the removal of the uterine lining and content.
Non-hormonal medications	Abnormal bleeding	This mainly includes nonsteroidal anti-inflammatory agents (NSAIDs).
Oral contraceptive pills	Abnormal bleeding, endometriosis	These can shrink endometrial tissue outside the uterus.
Progesterone intrauterine device (IUD)	Abnormal bleeding	

Hormonal medications	Abnormal bleeding, uterine fibroids, uterine prolapse	This may include progestins, GnRH agonists or oral contraceptives. These medications can shrink endometrial tissue outside the uterus.
Uterine artery embolization	Uterine fibroids	The uterine artery is surgically closed and stops blood flow to the fibroids.
Myomectomy	Uterine fibroids	Fibroids are removed without removing the uterus.
Laparotomy	Endometriosis	This surgical procedure removes endometrial tissue.
Kegel	Uterine prolapse	
Pessaries	Uterine prolapse	
Loop electrosurgical excision procedure (LEEP)	Precancerous cells in the cervix	This is a surgical procedure to eliminate precancerous cells without removing organs. However, the cells must be diagnosed early when conservative treatment is an option.

KNOWLEDGE IS POWER: LEARN ABOUT THE CONDITIONS THAT DON'T USUALLY REQUIRE A HYSTERECTOMY

Some gynecological conditions are serious and require a

hysterectomy (e.g., cancer). In contrast, some are relatively mild and can be managed non-surgically.

Then there is the gray area. The gray area is where your condition is not severe, but may require surgery because it's gotten out of hand. Below are conditions that typically don't require a hysterectomy, but sometimes do:

- Abnormal menstrual bleeding
- Uterine fibroids (unless severe or life-threatening)
- Endometriosis
- Dropped uterus
- Precancerous cervical lesions
- Chronic pelvic pain

You've already read about them in the previous chapter, so I won't elaborate here. Just keep these terms in mind as you make your decision.

THE PROS AND CONS OF A HYSTERECTOMY

Since everyone has a different reason for getting a hysterectomy, pros and cons may vary.

Below are the most noted benefits and risks of the surgery.

PROS

The top five advantages of a hysterectomy include:

1. If you have cancer, it can save your life.

A hysterectomy is often the best option to get rid of cancer. Leaving it inside or delaying the procedure can be risky because cancerous cells can spread quickly and become life-threatening.

2. It can improve your quality of life.

A hysterectomy can reduce pain from fibroids and endometriosis. However, your doctor must first investigate the pain and its exact cause. It can also boost energy levels and your overall health.

Women describe feeling like they got a new lease on life after the surgery. They report having no more pain, being in a better mood and feeling more productive.

> **Fair warning:** *Some women suffer from chronic pain even after a hysterectomy, while others develop new kinds of pain.*[16]

3. It can reduce excessive menstrual bleeding.

Excessive menstrual bleeding can lead to various complications and health risks. For example, you can quickly become anemic, suffer from low energy, feel weak and experience shortness of breath.

Excessive bleeding can also be a symptom of cancer and other severe complications, so getting it under control is liberating.

Remember that there are other less invasive options to reduce bleeding, so try those first.

4. **You won't need birth control.**

You can have no unwanted pregnancies. This can be a win for women who don't want hormonal birth control or intrauterine contraceptive devices.

5. **You'll be free from periods and feel more like yourself.**

Although a hysterectomy is a drastic step for stopping your periods, women who suffer from painful periods may benefit from a hysterectomy.

Removing your uterus will stop your menses, so it's also an ideal choice for trans men and non-binary individuals who don't want to get periods.

CONS

While many women live happy, normal lives after the surgery, there *are* some things you should be aware of. I'll start with the biggest downside for most people:

1. **You can have no further children in your uterus, although surrogacy may still be an option.**

Removing the uterus removes the possibility of getting pregnant. If you can keep your ovaries, these will produce eggs, and you'll have the option to have a biological baby through surrogacy.

2. It interferes with your hormones.

A hysterectomy, including an oophorectomy (removal of the ovaries), may affect hormone levels or trigger early menopause. Side effects you can expect are vaginal atrophy, urinary leakage, weight gain and loss of libido.

3. Possible vaginal problems.

If the cervix is removed, there is a risk of problems at the top of the vagina. Other possible complications include infection, delayed wound healing following surgery, and prolapse in subsequent years.[17]

4. Ovarian failure.

Partial hysterectomies (removing the uterus but not the ovaries) may impair blood flow to the ovaries and affect hormonal balance.[18]

Even if one or both ovaries are intact, you may still experience menopausal symptoms earlier than expected, and you're twice as likely to suffer ovarian failure.[19]

5. Potential organ prolapse of the vagina, bladder or other organs.

The organs of your reproductive system support each other like interlocked puzzle pieces. When one or more of them are removed, the support is compromised.

This can put too much pressure on your pelvic floor muscles because they now have a more significant role in holding the organs in place.

If these muscles and ligaments weaken, the pelvic organs (womb, bladder, bowels) may shift downward and out of their normal position, creating a vaginal bulge. This is known as prolapse and affects nearly 40% of women after a hysterectomy.[20]

6. Early menopause.

A radical or total hysterectomy puts you in menopause immediately. However, other types of hysterectomies, where your ovaries are retained, also cause early menopause, although not right away.

Hormone replacement therapy combats this to some extent. But it also has severe side effects, such as heart attack, stroke and breast cancer, so long-term use is not recommended.

7. It puts you at high risk for mental and physical diseases.

> *"A study of females who underwent hysterectomy without ovary removal from 1980–2002 found a 6.6% higher risk for new depression diagnoses and a 4.7% higher risk for anxiety diagnoses in the 20 years following their surgery."*[25]
>
> *FLETCHER, 2023C*

A hysterectomy can cause:

- 1.3 times increased risk of lipid abnormalities[21]
- 6% increased risk of coronary (heart) artery disease[22]
- 4.6-fold increased risk of congestive heart failure
- 2.5-fold increased risk of coronary artery disease
- 1% increased risk of prolapse 3 years after a hysterectomy and up to 15% increase 15 years post-surgery (Alkatout et al., n.d.)[23]
- 26% increased risk of depression in women over age 35[24]
- 47% increased risk of depression for women under 35 years old
- 22% increased risk for anxiety in women over 35 years old
- 45% increased risk for anxiety in women under 35 years old

8. There are possible surgical complications.

Surgeries always hold some risk, no matter how safe the procedure is. Surgical complications related to a hysterectomy include:[26]

- The nerves near the uterus may be damaged during a hysterectomy, which can lead to stress incontinence (leaking urine).
- Complications from anesthesia

- Bleeding

- Ureter damage

- Bladder or bowel damage

- Infection

- Blood clots

COMPARING THE PROS AND CONS OF THE TYPES OF HYSTERECTOMIES			
	Pros	**Cons**	**When is it advised?**
Total hysterectomy	Gets rid of the problem. Decreases pain and discomfort.	Menopause, surgical complications, no more biological kids.	Cancer in one organ, risk of cancer spreading.
Subtotal hysterectomy	Fixes the issue with minimal organ removal.	Since the cervix is left in place, there's still a risk of cervical cancer developing.	Fibroids, endometriosis, or problems contained in specific areas.
Total hysterectomy with bilateral salpingo-oophorectomy	Relieves symptoms and improves the quality of life.	Immediate menopause.	Family history of ovarian cancer.

Radical hysterectomy	Fixes the issue and gets rid of the pain.	Unable to get pregnant. Unable to have children even via surrogacy. Early menopause.	When cancer treatments have not been successful or are not suitable.

WHEN SHOULD YOU CONSIDER GETTING A HYSTERECTOMY?

Now that you know the possible pros and cons of this procedure, let's cover some situations when getting a hysterectomy may be considered[26]:

WHEN ALL OTHER OPTIONS HAVE FAILED

Medications, lifestyle changes and minor surgeries don't work for everyone. They didn't work for me. So don't be reluctant to schedule a hysterectomy if you've tried everything else.

IF YOU DON'T MIND PERMANENT BIRTH CONTROL

If you already have children, don't want kids, or don't want any more, a hysterectomy may be feasible if other approaches have failed to resolve your condition.

FAMILY HISTORY OF CANCER

You can get a hysterectomy if you have a family history of uterine, cervical or ovarian cancer.

Angelina Jolie had a laparoscopic bilateral salpingo-oophorectomy because of her genetic risk of uterine cancer.[27]

IMMEDIATE TREATMENT

You should schedule a hysterectomy if you have a life-threatening illness like cancer or excessive bleeding. Trying less invasive treatments might not be an option for you.

I know that was a lot. This chapter has a lot of dark content. Let's take a deep breath together.

Here's a recap of the main topics we covered.

- Don't be afraid to ask questions. The more you know, the more equipped you'll be for this tough decision.

- Identify the root problem that's causing your symptoms. Understand your treatment options. Try them first instead of rushing into a hysterectomy.

- The biggest pros of hysterectomy are that it can save your life and improve your quality of life by alleviating pain and reducing excessive bleeding.

- The cons of hysterectomy include surgical complications, permanent birth control, physical and mental problems, hormonal imbalances, early menopause and vaginal issues.

- Don't hesitate to schedule the surgery if all else has failed, you have a family history of cancer, or you need immediate treatment.

Although I've talked about the pros and cons at length, it's okay if you still have questions.

Answers can provide peace of mind and help you solidify your decision. If you're considering a hysterectomy but need more information before committing, the next chapter will clarify these things for you.

Chapter 4

"If you don't ask the right questions, you don't get the right answers. A question asked in the right way often points to its own answer. Asking questions is the ABC of diagnosis. Only the inquiring mind solves problems."

EDWARD HODNETT

Before my procedure, I had thoroughly researched the complications, side effects and benefits of getting a hysterectomy. Yet, I encountered many unexpected challenges afterward — a testament that we can always learn something new.

Not only are hysterectomies complex, but there are different types, surgical approaches, patient presentations, indications, risks and outcomes.

Let's dig into the FAQs on what to expect before, during and after surgery.

BEFORE SURGERY

The time before surgery is often nerve-racking and filled with cumbersome pre-op directives. To prepare for the operation, here are some precautions to keep in mind.

1. Can I smoke before having a hysterectomy?

Although you *can* smoke, it is preferred not to do so. Smoking introduces harmful chemicals into the body that stay in your lungs and respiratory tract long after you've finished the cigarette.

These chemicals increase the likelihood of respiratory infections, pneumonia, heart problems, anesthetic complications, surgical complications, a weaker immune system, lung collapse and longer recovery time.

It's best to quit smoking as early as possible. Quitting approximately eight weeks before your surgery can cut the risk of complications by 48%.[27]

2. Can I eat and drink before surgery?

Doctors recommend not eating or drinking 6-12 hours before surgery. However, the anesthesiologist may recommend a shorter duration of 4 hours, depending on your surgery.

Having food or water in your stomach can be dangerous during the operation. There's a risk of the food coming up (as vomit) and going into the respiratory tract and lungs while your reflexes and muscle control are compromised under anesthesia.[28]

You can drink clear fluids, such as water, black coffee and apple juice, up to four hours before.

3. What foods should I avoid before surgery?

If you're going under general anesthesia, you should avoid nuts, high-fiber foods, fruits, whole grains, fish, omega-3 and milk; white carbs, such as rice and pasta; and spices, such as garlic and ginger.

Up to two weeks before surgery, refrain from foods, spices and supplements containing omega-3, garlic or ginger.

These foods digest slowly and may affect blood clotting, making surgery challenging.

4. Should I lose weight before the hysterectomy?

Ideally, yes. You should try to lose as much weight as possible before the procedure to improve your outcome. Losing weight isn't easy, especially when you're not feeling well, but it has several benefits, including reduced risk of complications during and after surgery.

Being overweight or obese increases the chance of surgical complications, such as infections, blood clots, delayed wound healing, breathing problems and heart attack.

5. Is combining a hysterectomy with another procedure, such as a tummy tuck, possible?

Yes, it is possible to combine a hysterectomy with a tummy tuck. Benefits include cost savings, fewer surgeries and quicker recovery, in some cases.

While the operation is relatively safe, it's not recommended for everyone. A 2012 study evaluated 65 women who combined both surgeries and found that 32% (20) had complications.[29]

Your combined surgery takes 4-6 hours. The longer you're under anesthesia, the greater your risk – but the better your health, the lower your risk.

It's best to talk to your doctor, evaluate your options, and review your insurance and costs before scheduling both surgeries together.

6. Why is one type of hysterectomy procedure recommended over other types?

Your doctor will recommend the safest procedure most likely to fix the problem and with the quickest recovery.

For example, if your surgeon believes a vaginal hysterectomy will resolve your issue, they'll recommend it. However, if they feel it'll cause unnecessary complications, they'll suggest something else.

Similarly, a radical hysterectomy is usually the last option your doctor will recommend *unless* it's your best option.

7. What are the effects of removing the cervix from the body versus leaving it intact?

The effects of removing the cervix versus keeping it depend on the gynecological issue that prompted you to schedule surgery.

Your surgeon may remove it to prevent recurrent cervical cancer, for instance. However, leaving the cervix can cause continued cyclical vaginal bleeding, painful periods and urine leakage.[30]

Both options have advantages and disadvantages, but check with your doctor for clarification on which benefits your condition.

8. Which organs and structures are removed?

Your doctor can remove one or all organs of your reproductive system, depending on the type of procedure.

(Feel free to revisit Chapter 1 to review which structures are removed in each type of hysterectomy.)

9. What is left in my body after a total hysterectomy?

A total hysterectomy removes the uterus and cervix. So, you will retain your ovaries, fallopian tubes, cervix and vagina.

However, if your procedure is paired with other types, such as a total hysterectomy with salpingo-oophorectomy, you'll have fewer organs after the operation.

10. Will I get visible scars from the surgery?

The size, location and visibility of your scars depend on the type of hysterectomy you receive.

An abdominal hysterectomy leaves the largest scar, thanks to a 6–8-inch cut that runs layers deep and spans the abdomen horizontally or vertically.

A vaginal hysterectomy does not leave a visible scar because the incisions occur within the vagina.

During a laparoscopic hysterectomy, you'll receive 3-6 small cuts in different locations on the abdomen, with one near your belly button. These leave little scars, much less visible than those from an abdominal procedure.

During a robotic-assisted procedure, you'll get 4-5 tiny incisions, which leave scars that are similar to those from a laparoscopic hysterectomy.

As technology progresses, single-site hysterectomy is another option. It uses a robot to access the reproductive organs through your belly button.

You'll get a tiny incision within the navel. The incision is covered after the procedure, so there's barely any scar from it.

DURING SURGERY AND YOUR HOSPITAL STAY

Here are answers to frequently asked questions about the experience during the procedure and hospital stay.

1. How long will the surgery take?

A hysterectomy takes 1-2 hours. However, the duration can increase if there are complications.

2. Will I be completely naked during the surgery? If so, for how long?

Not always, although it is a possibility.

Surgeons will remove your hospital gown and put a sterilized drape over you during surgery. Depending on the surgical approach, the drape will have holes to give surgeons access to the abdomen or vagina.

Once the drape is placed, you'll only be exposed around the areas where the surgeons are working.[31] Nurses usually cover you up as soon as the surgery ends.

If you're fully naked, it'll only be between when your gown is removed and the drape is placed.

Some hospitals give you the right to choose certain things regarding modesty and privacy in the operating room. If you have this opportunity, communicate your preferences to stay as dressed as possible during the surgery.

3. How long will I remain in the hospital?

The duration of your hospital stay depends on your health and the surgical approach. You'll generally remain in the hospital for up to five days after an open abdominal hysterectomy. However, you can be released on the same day or within 24 hours after a laparoscopic procedure.

4. Will I be independent in caring for my personal needs and hygiene at the hospital? If not, who should I ask for support?

You won't be conscious enough to take care of your needs immediately after the surgery, so a designated nurse will take care of you.

Once the anesthesia wears off, you can take care of *only those* personal needs that don't require too much movement or energy. You'll slowly return to full function and go to the bathroom alone, take a walk, change your clothes and so on.

You can ask the hospital staff to help you if you need anything. Additionally, family or friends who are staying with you can help too.

5. **How long before the surgery will I have to go under anesthesia?**

You'll go under anesthesia immediately before the surgery.

6. **Can I take my regular medication on the day of surgery and while at the hospital?**

Only sometimes. This depends on the type of medication.

Medications that require food can cause stomach irritation and nausea if you take them without food. (Remember you're not allowed solid food after midnight before the day of operation.)

Because aspirin products can cause bleeding problems, they should be avoided a week before surgery.

Blood pressure medication can affect your cardiac function and blood pressure when you're under anesthesia, so be cautious of those. However, your doctor may instruct you to continue taking it on the morning of your surgery.

That's why it's important to share your list of medications with the doctor and get confirmation on which ones to take or avoid.

7. **Can I wear any jewelry?**

You're often not allowed to wear jewelry (including piercings) during surgery. Jewelry is unsafe because electricity can pass through it and burn you if the surgical staff uses a defibrillator to shock your heart into rhythm.

It can also get in the way of the procedure, even if it's not at the surgery site.

AFTER SURGERY

NAUSEA, BLOATING AND GAS

1. Will I be nauseous after the surgery?

Yes, there is a high likelihood that you'll wake up nauseous after the surgery. Research shows that most women undergoing spinal anesthesia suffer postoperative nausea and vomiting.[32]

2. When will my stomach bloating go down?

Bloating after surgery is normal. It's a side effect of anesthesia, constipation, fluid retention or damage to the lymphatic system.[33] It usually goes away within a few days or a couple of weeks.

Eating fiber, getting enough fluids, moving around, and taking stool softeners can help.

3. How long will it take constipation and gas to go away?

Constipation and gas last a few days to a week after a hysterectomy. Anesthesia and painkillers containing opioids can cause constipation. The quicker you receive treatment to alleviate it, the sooner you'll feel better.

Most women have their first bowel movement within five days post-op.

Your doctor may prescribe stool softeners and fiber laxatives to ease bowel movements. If you're severely constipated, stimulant laxatives and suppositories may provide faster relief.

BLEEDING

1. Is it normal to bleed after a hysterectomy?

Yes, bleeding is common after the surgery.

Light bleeding can continue for a few days to several weeks as the tissues heal. It's vital to use sanitary pads instead of tampons to prevent infection.

If there's heavy bleeding or the blood is bright red and accompanied by a foul odor or large clots, contact your doctor immediately. These are not normal.

2. Can you bleed if you just have your ovaries?

Yes, you can bleed a little if your uterus is removed, but you still have ovaries and cervix. There is some endometrial tissue in the cervix as well. It can shed and bleed similarly to periods (but with less flow intensity) when the estrogen from the ovaries act on it.[34]

If the cervix and uterus are completely removed, you will not bleed even if your ovaries are intact.

3. Will I still have PMS after my hysterectomy?

Yes, you may experience PMS and bloating if you still have your ovaries, but the severity is often shorter and less intense. However, if your ovaries are removed, you will no longer experience PMS, and menopause will kick in.

4. What does it mean if I'm bleeding years after my hysterectomy?

Bleeding years after a total hysterectomy is not common. It could indicate benign growths, such as a polyp, cancerous cells damaging the tissues in the vagina or nearby areas, or colon or bladder issues.

You should see a doctor immediately if it happens. However, if you see brown or dark discharge but not blood, it could be due to an infection or rupture inside your vagina.

5. What would cause bleeding after a hysterectomy?

Some causes of bleeding are atrophic vaginitis (thinning and drying of the vaginal walls due to low estrogen), vault endometriosis, fistula around the bowel, pelvic hematoma, vaginal cuff tear, hemorrhage and cancer.[35]

CARE

1. How do I dress my wounds?

Wounds from an open abdominal hysterectomy require the most care. It is crucial to keep them clean and dry to prevent infection. Your surgeon may recommend using sterile gauze or dressings, which should be changed regularly to cover the wound.

Wash the wound with mild soap and warm water; watch out for smelly discharge, blood or pus.

2. When can I take a shower or bathe after surgery?

You can shower 48 hours after surgery. Pat your incisions dry as soon as possible. Avoid soaking or getting the area too wet until the cut is completely healed and the sutures or staples are out, so no baths for a couple of weeks.

Some surgeons use absorbable stitches, so don't be alarmed if your doctor doesn't advise you to wait for the stitches to come out.

SLEEP

Can I sleep on my stomach after a hysterectomy?

You should avoid sleeping on your stomach for a few weeks after the surgery. Doctors recommend the same for abdominal and laparoscopic hysterectomies.

Sleeping on your stomach can put unnecessary pressure on the wound site, spine and hips.

It's best to sleep on your back in a semi-sitting position. You can use pillows to help you maintain that position or sleep on a recliner. You can also sleep on your side with pillows between your legs and beneath your stomach to provide additional support and keep you from rolling.

PAIN

1. How long will it take to heal after a hysterectomy? Will I be in pain?

In addition to your physical state, your mental, emotional and sexual well-being should be considered as well. It takes 2-6 weeks of proper rest to heal, but this time frame varies from person to person.

You may experience physical and emotional pain during recovery, such as pain from the surgery or feeling a sense of loss emotionally and mentally.

2. It's been months since my hysterectomy. Why am I still in pain?

Post-surgical chronic pain is unfortunately common after a hysterectomy. It can be due to several factors like intense pelvic pain before the surgery and high levels of unmanaged pain after the procedure.

Differences in pain tolerance and medication response also influence chronic pain duration. The good news is that the pain intensity goes down for most women over time.

3. Why do my back, hips and joints hurt?

Reasons for back, hip and joint pain after the procedure include pelvic floor muscle spasms/hypertonia, scar tissue from the procedure, infections, direct trauma to the pelvic area, being in the lithotomy position (in stirrups) during surgery, and decreased blood to the local nerves and muscles.

Treatment often includes medications, physical therapy and exercise. The pain may not go away quickly, and you may have to find ways to deal with it. Some women experience such pain only occasionally after extraneous activity or emotional stress.

4. Will it hurt to sit after a hysterectomy?

Your pelvic floor muscles must support the reproductive organs after the reshuffling post-surgery. This puts them under a lot of pressure, and if they're not strong enough, they can spasm. When that happens, it can hurt to sit or stand because the organs push down, but the muscles don't adjust accordingly.

Applying a heating pad and practicing Kegel exercises can help.

5. Why does it burn when I use the bathroom?

A burning sensation while emptying the bladder is a symptom of a urinary tract infection. Unfortunately, these are common after hospital stays, especially if you had a catheter.

Medications and plenty of fluids should resolve this.

6. **How long will it take to stop hurting when I laugh, cough or sneeze following surgery?**

It'll take roughly six weeks to cough without feeling your entire abdomen shake or hurt. Rest assured, the force won't be enough to break abdominal sutures.

You can try hugging a pillow, pressing down on the incision site with your hands, or bending slightly forward while coughing, sneezing or laughing to ease the pain.

SEXUAL INTERCOURSE

1. **How soon after surgery can I resume sexual activities?**

You can return to non-penetrative sexual activities whenever you're comfortable, but you should not insert anything (including a tampon) into your vagina for at least six weeks post-surgery. This is after your wounds have healed and you are no longer bleeding or have a vaginal discharge.

2. **Will sexual intercourse hurt after a hysterectomy?**

Sex isn't painful for most women who enjoyed pain-free intercourse before surgery. However, watch out for vaginal dryness, which can be painful. If you have difficulty getting wet, lubricating creams can help.

3. **Will my partner be able to tell that I've had a hysterectomy during intimacy?**

No, sex won't feel different for your partner after your procedure. The vagina is usually intact after most hysterectomies.

ACTIVITIES

1. How much weight can I lift after surgery?

You can only carry 10-20 pounds (anywhere from a gallon of milk to a half-filled bag of groceries) for six weeks after the procedure.

Gradually increase the weight as you regain your strength, but use proper posture so you don't put too much stress on your incisions while lifting.

2. Can I do my laundry, vacuum or bend down?

You should refrain from heavy housework in the first six weeks. This includes doing the laundry and vacuuming.

Bending down is also discouraged, as it puts pressure on your incisions. The timeline is typically 2-8 weeks, but check with your doctor at your next checkup.

If you must bend to pick something up, sit down first or squat down slowly at the knees instead of bending your back.

3. Can I take the stairs?

Yes, you can go up and down the stairs after your surgery or when you're ready.

Start slowly by initially putting both feet on the same step, supporting your climb, and not carrying any objects that may affect your balance or add more weight.

You can resume regular stair climbing roughly six weeks post-surgery.

4. When can I start driving again?

You can get behind the wheel 2-6 weeks after the procedure. Although this is the recommended time, you should only drive if you are no longer sedated or using prescription opioids.

You should also be comfortable wearing a seatbelt, looking over your shoulder, driving the car and making emergency stops.

5. How soon after surgery can I exercise?

You can start walking slowly on the same day after the procedure. Increase the duration and add light exercises, such as deep breathing, pelvic exercises and gentle stretching, until you have your doctor's approval to return to regular activities. This may take 4-6 weeks.

Exercise can put pressure on your stomach while you're healing. For example, the pressure from your legs while doing a leg press can compress your belly. Intense ab exercises can strain your abdomen and pelvic floor.

Watch out for these issues and pace yourself. Always listen to your body, check with your doctor, and remember that rest is necessary for recovery.

6. When can I return to work?

Most women can return to work within 6-8 weeks after

surgery, but you may need more or less time, depending on your vocation.

7. What happens if I overdo it after a hysterectomy?

You may experience intense pain, vaginal bleeding or discharge longer than a few weeks, oozing incisions, and risk internal damage if you do too much too soon after your procedure.

That's why it's crucial to get all the rest you can. Your body goes through a lot and needs time to heal.

OTHER

1. Can I have kids after a hysterectomy, and will I still have periods?

You can't get pregnant after a hysterectomy because you no longer have a uterus. However, you can have kids through surrogacy if your ovaries are intact and healthy because they can produce eggs.

You can also have regular menstrual cycles after a hysterectomy if your ovaries are intact. Still, you won't bleed because of the absence of a uterus, but you can bleed if you have a partial uterus.

A rare complication after a hysterectomy is ectopic pregnancy, where the fetus begins to form outside of the uterus. It happens if you're still fertile, so you may have to use contraception even after a hysterectomy.[36]

2. Will I gain or lose weight after the surgery?

Many women gain weight after the procedure, while others lose weight. Menopause, or the onset of menopausal symptoms, is the biggest reason for weight gain because it's associated with hormonal imbalances.

Weight loss after a hysterectomy can be due to cancer or a similar underlying condition that requires immediate medical attention, but it's not always the case.

3. Will a hysterectomy make me age faster?

Yes, a hysterectomy causes menopause or puts you in a premenopausal state. This produces physical and metabolic changes in the body that are often associated with aging.

4. Will I still need to have pelvic exams?

Yes, pelvic exams are still recommended, even after a hysterectomy, but their frequency may reduce to every 3-5 years. However, your doctor may request yearly exams to rule out cancer if there's a genetic risk.

Pelvic exams check for cancers in the reproductive tract, new fibroids or cysts in the ovaries, and the health of the rectum, vagina, fallopian tubes, ovaries, cervix and uterus.

This covers the most frequently asked questions about a hysterectomy. I wish I had all these answers before my surgery. Hopefully, you can now make a more informed decision before moving forward with yours.

Let's do a quick review.

- Don't eat anything at least 6 hours before surgery.

- Try to quit smoking as early as possible.

- If you're overweight, losing weight before surgery can improve the outcome.

- You can combine your hysterectomy with another procedure, such as a tummy tuck.

- A hysterectomy takes 1-2 hours. You may remain in the hospital for 24 hours or up to 5 days.

- You can request that you're covered up as much as possible during the operation.

- Nurses, family and friends can help you with your personal needs while hospitalized.

- Consult your doctor about taking regular medications before surgery.

- Bloating and feeling nauseous are normal after the operation. They usually go away within a few days or a couple of weeks.

- Constipation and gas last a few days to a week after a hysterectomy.

- You should expect light bleeding after the procedure, but you won't have periods afterward.

- Bleeding years after a total hysterectomy is not typical. You should get it checked out.

- Clean your wound with mild soap and warm water

and keep it dry until it heals. Take showers, but avoid baths for a few weeks after the surgery.

- Don't sleep on your stomach for the first few weeks after the procedure.

- Your back and hips can hurt after the operation. Sitting can also be painful due to spasms in the pelvic floor muscles.

- It takes about 6 weeks to cough, sneeze and laugh without pain.

- You can have sexual intercourse after 6 weeks. No, it won't hurt in most cases. Your partner can't tell the difference.

- You can carry 10-20 pounds during the first 6 weeks. Use the stairs, but go slowly.

- Return to work in 6-8 weeks and drive in 2-6 weeks or when you feel up to it.

- You can't get pregnant after the procedure. Yes, surrogacy is an option if the ovaries are intact.

- A hysterectomy may make you age faster and possibly gain weight.

Now that we've tackled the burning questions, the next question is how to best prepare once you've decided to proceed with the surgery.

Chapter 5

"The will to succeed is important, but what's more important is the will to prepare."

BOBBY KNIGHT

Y ou may feel sicker as you get closer to surgery. You may experience more bleeding, pain, loss of appetite and nausea, depending on why you're having the surgery. If you've lost a lot of blood, you may also require a blood transfusion.

Additionally, you may have mixed emotions about the procedure and your outcome.

You may be **fearful** about how you'll feel afterward. I remember being afraid that I would never be the same. Not be at the same fitness level or have periods. *Yes, periods.* I was shocked to feel this way, especially since they had made me miserable most of my life.

I was also afraid of being menopausal, that the surgery wouldn't eliminate my pain, and that I'd be unable to maintain my weight.

You may feel **hopeful** that you won't be in agony anymore or that the surgery will remove cancerous cells from your body or help with pelvic prolapse.

You may also feel **relieved** to finally get a chance to rest after surgery, especially if you've been tired for so long.

You may feel **sad, anxious or alone** because you've never had kids or want more kids, but won't be able to after the procedure, or like the choice is being taken away. You may also feel **less of a woman** without your organs.

You may feel that you'll **never be the same,** that **sex** won't feel the same, life won't be the same, your **family and friends** won't know what you're going through or understand, that you'll be out of work for too long or even lose your **job** for being on extended leave, that you'll **gain weight,** or go into **immediate menopause** and start feeling all the symptoms of it.

You may feel **overwhelmed** and that you need more time to organize everything.

You may feel **out of control** and too **dependent** on others.

You may **worry** about who will care for your children or manage the chores when you're out of commission.

You may wonder if the surgery will be successful and if you'll make it through alive.

Getting a handle on these emotions can impact your physical, mental and emotional health.

Please know that these feelings are normal and that everyone manages them differently. I experienced many of these emotions too, but it does get better.

There is a light at the end of the tunnel.

So, *how* do you deal with all these emotions?

Preparing for the days ahead can curb some of the anxiety and negative thoughts that may be surfacing now that you've decided to move forward with the procedure.

Setting up a support system before surgery and arming yourself with knowledge can also help.

Below, you'll find tips on what to do at different stages of your journey to deal with these emotions.

PREPARING FOR SURGERY: HANDY CHECKLISTS FOR A BETTER EXPERIENCE

I'll share recommendations and practical steps for setting up your home and support systems for those first few days at home and exactly what you will need to do, even if you're alone (divorced/separated/single) or don't have kids or anyone nearby.

TWO MONTHS BEFORE

Surgery is not just a physical ordeal. It's a mental one, too. So, start by **managing your mindset** and regulating your mood. Here are some things you can try:

- Deep breathing and relaxation exercises
- Yoga
- Brisk walks
- Medication
- Spiritual healing and spending time with God

Try to **stop smoking and cultivate healthy habits,** especially those you can sustain after surgery. These may include exercising regularly, adding healthy green vegetables and fruits to your diet, and keeping a good sleep schedule.

Small adjustments can significantly change your outcome.

Find a good **mental health professional** if you can afford one. They can offer great solutions and a safe space to share your fears and concerns.

You can also **journal how you're feeling,** which can help you reduce stress, manage anxiety, cope with depression, boost emotional intelligence, and express your raw, unfiltered thoughts. Journaling was primarily how I made it through the rough patches.

Surround yourself with **genuine and positive people.** Their attitude is contagious even when life looks bleak. It's easy to fall into a rabbit hole of negative thoughts and worst-case scenarios when you're going through a tough time, and positive people can pull you out of it.

Create a **support system** through your family, friends and neighbors. Tell them what's happening with you and what you need help with, then be open to their support.

You can also find support groups online or in your local community of women going through a similar situation. Hysterectomy veterans can give you perspective, letting you know that most of your worries will never materialize.

Reduce stressors in your life where you can. For example, if you have too much responsibility at work, try to step back for your health.

Hire house help or ask your support system for assistance if you can't afford it. Adult kids can handle chores around the home, such as grocery shopping, vacuuming, doing the dishes, laundry, etc.

Identify which aspects of the day drain you, then work to eliminate the most significant stressors.

ONE MONTH BEFORE

Check your **medical insurance and deductibles** and determine if you can make payment arrangements to cover surgery costs.

Keep a financial buffer in case you need more tests, your hospital stay is extended, or something unexpected happens. Share these details with a trusted partner or friend (if one is available) so they can manage affairs while you're incapacitated.

Have your primary and secondary insurance information ready for the pre-registration for surgery. Update your **emergency contact** information and share any changes with a confidant.

Speak with your doctor about what to expect during the procedure and recovery time, including:

- What supplements (and herbal products) to take and stop. For example, too much chamomile, vitamin E, ginger and garlic can cause bleeding problems. List all supplements and herbs you regularly take and check if you can safely continue consuming them a month before the surgery.

- Share any medications you are taking and ask if any need to change before surgery (e.g., blood thinners).

- What over-the-counter medication or scripts you can get before the surgery.

- If you should change your current medication routine and when.

- If you'll need special supplies or equipment when you're discharged. If so, can you get them now to prepare your home?

Ask what **limitations** you'll have following surgery and how long the recovery period will last.

These limitations can be physical, such as how much weight you can carry and your sleeping posture. Also, ask when you can return to work, sex, exercise and strenuous activity.

Create a timeline on paper or your computer with that information. Knowing when you can return to the activities you love can motivate you to power through the tough times and make them more bearable.

Have charcoal pills, laxatives and a heating pad on standby. You can get these before the procedure.

Invest in a body pillow and cold compress to improve your rest quality and manage swelling.

Get as **fit and healthy** as you can.

- Try to stop or reduce smoking to prevent respiratory infections.

- Exercise daily, even if it's a light walk.

- Try to lose some weight if you are overweight.

P.S. If you need help with any of these, consider getting a health coach or professional guidance.

Schedule your **medical leave at work** (if applicable) and fill out any necessary paperwork. Be prepared to take 2-6 weeks off.

Have the surgeon **check your iron levels**. If you're anemic, you may need an iron supplement or a blood transfusion before surgery. This is an essential preparatory step because many gynecological problems, such as excessive menstrual bleeding and fibroids, may cause severe anemia and affect the surgery.

Find a friend, neighbor or family member who can drive you home after you're discharged or help with chores during your recovery.

ONE WEEK BEFORE

Shop for necessities (toiletries, food, pet food, etc.) to cover the first three weeks post-surgery. Stock your pantry with light and healthy snacks and quick meals.

You can **prepare multiple meals** that will last a few weeks and freeze them for easy reheating. Alternatively, a reliable food delivery service or someone from your support system may be able to assist.

Some healthy post-surgery food options include:

- Soups and healthy broths

- Fresh fruit and vegetables, especially those rich in vitamins A and C. These include green leafy vegetables, cruciferous vegetables, and fruits like pineapple, cantaloupe, citrus fruits, juices and tomato juice.

- Healthy smoothies. Ideally, make them sugar-free. You can freeze fully prepared smoothies or cut and freeze the ingredients to put in a blender when you want to make the drink.

- Lean meat

- Eggs

- Nuts and seeds. Only eat a handful of these. Although they're loaded with healthy fats, consuming too many can contribute to weight gain.

Avoid high-fat meats, processed and oily foods, too many

spices, dairy products, gassy foods and drinks, and sugary sweets that increase constipation and gas.

Reorganize your room and living space for your recovery time. This may include putting things within reach and moving your bedroom to the first floor if you'd rather not use the stairs.

Have a few good books, magazines or movies lined up, as you may not be able to move around much. Such entertainment will be a welcome distraction.

Cross off as many chores and to-dos from your list as possible or outsource them for a few weeks.

Pack loose clothing and a soft pillow for the ride back home from the hospital. A pillow will be your best friend. Don't leave it behind.

Pack some **toiletries for your time at the hospital**. You can also load up fun podcasts or keep a book to pass the time.

Confirm you have someone to take you home or help with chores and pets.

Have Hibiclens or an **antiseptic soap** on standby. Keeping your wounds clean and infection-free is vital for recovery.

Follow your doctor's advice for medication on the days leading up to surgery. Set up reminders on your phone so you don't miss a dose.

If you haven't already, pick up your **pre-filled prescriptions** and put them in an accessible location, preferably beside your bed.

Drink plenty of water to reduce constipation. Place a water dispenser next to your bed, or fill small to medium-sized bottles with water and store them nearby so you won't have to get up to refill them.

Verify that your doctor and anesthesiologist know the medications and supplements you're taking. Put the list in an email or take a photo in case you misplace them.

You may need a medical assessment a few days before the hysterectomy. Find out if or when it's required.

THE DAY BEFORE

Keep practicing your **breathing exercises and relaxation drills** to calm your nerves. Invite a friend or partner to keep you company if you need the distraction. Trust that you have everything sorted for the big day.

Pack your **hospital bag** with the following:

- Travel-sized toiletries
- Sanitary pads for post-surgery bleeds
- Lip-salve, lotions
- Cough drops (for post-surgery sore throat)
- Extra socks if your feet get cold
- Something to read or do before and after surgery

- Notepad and pen to jot down notes

- Loose, comfy clothing (including a soft bra). Avoid anything that will restrict or chafe your abdomen.

- Pillow while in the hospital and for the ride home

- Cellphone and charger

These are just necessities. You can add more items as needed, such as your prescription glasses.

Follow the **pre-op team's directions** for body and hair care. You may need to bathe with an antiseptic soap the day before and the morning of surgery.

You may also be instructed to eat a light breakfast and lunch, followed by clear fluids the day before. If you need to take a bowel cleansing solution, take it on this day.

Write down important notes on your **medical, surgery and family health history**. Also, keep a **list of your meds** on hand to provide to the hospital.

Leave your **jewelry** at home; only keep essential items in your hospital bag.

Being on your menstrual cycle won't delay the surgery. Many women, including myself, have a hysterectomy due to excessive bleeding and prolonged periods.

However, if you're sick, you may need to reschedule, depending on the procedure's urgency and how sick you are. Your doctor will decide if the surgery needs to be postponed.

Any illness that affects your respiratory system, like pneumonia or the flu, may delay the procedure, however.

Minor problems like sniffles shouldn't be a problem, but tell your doctor if you're not feeling well. Having jitters and sweating from anxiety is also not a concern.

MIND OVER MATTER. THIS IS JUST AS MUCH A MENTAL BATTLE AS A PHYSICAL ONE.

You can't do much about the physical pain and issues, but you can take steps to manage your mental health. Do your best to focus on positive things and a good outcome.

Here are a few tips to keep your mind off the surgery:

- Have a few **movies, books, board games** or something distracting and uplifting lined up.

- Organize a **tranquilizer** up front if you feel you may need one. Consult with your doctor to see if it's safe to take and when.

- Try **belly breathing.** It's an excellent way to manage your breathing and slow it down when your mind starts spiraling or if you're hyperventilating.

- Use a **positive mantra or affirmations**. These are more powerful than most people realize. Repeating them can ease your mind and put you in an optimistic mood.

  A few include:

◊   I will wake up quickly and feel refreshed after surgery.

◊   I trust in my body's ability to heal and accept the treatment.

◊   I trust my doctor and the healthcare team to use their skills for my good.

- **Visualize a successful surgery.** Convincing yourself that you'll be fine afterward can boost your mood.

Don't stress about remembering everything I've mentioned in this chapter. Instead, use the checklists on the following pages to check off items you've completed and sort the ones left.

Great! You now know how to prepare your mind, body, finances and home for the procedure.

You won't feel too anxious if you know what to expect on surgery day. We'll cover that next.

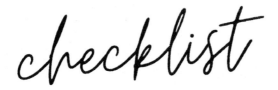

checklist

2 Months Before Surgery

- ☐ Check your medical insurance and deductibles
- ☐ Keep a financial buffer for additional costs
- ☐ Have your insurance information ready
- ☐ Update your emergency contact information
- ☐ Speak with your doctor about what to expect during surgery
- ☐ Ask what type of limitations you'll have
- ☐ Schedule your medical leave
- ☐ Try to quit smoking
- ☐ Try to lose weight if you're overweight

checklist

1 Month Before Surgery

- [ ] Manage your mindset and mood
- [ ] Journal how you're feeling
- [ ] Cultivate healing lifestyle habits
- [ ] Surround yourself with positive people
- [ ] Have a support system in place
- [ ] Identity and reduce stressors
- [ ] Get charcoal pills, laxatives and a heating pad
- [ ] Invest in a body pillow and cold compress
- [ ] Check your iron levels

checklist

1 Week Before Surgery

- [ ] Shop for all your necessities
- [ ] Prepare recovery meals and freeze them
- [ ] Reorganize your room and living space
- [ ] Line up some good books or movies
- [ ] Cross off chores and to-dos or outsource them
- [ ] Pack some toiletries for your time at the hospital
- [ ] Confirm that someone is available to drive you to and from the hospital for surgery
- [ ] Have Hibiclens or an antiseptic soap on standby
- [ ] Pick up your pre-filled prescriptions
- [ ] Jot down a list of your medications and supplements for the hospital staff
- [ ] Check if you need a medical assessment before surgery and schedule it

checklist

1 Day Before Surgery

- ☐ Practice meditation exercises and relaxation drills
- ☐ Shower/bathe as instructed by the doctor
- ☐ Eat a light breakfast and lunch
- ☐ Take a bowel cleansing oral solution
- ☐ Write down your medical, surgery and family health history
- ☐ Email or take a photo of your list of medications and supplements in case you misplace it
- ☐ Leave jewelry at home
- ☐ Recite a positive mantra or affirmation
- ☐ Try belly breathing
- ☐ Pack your hospital bag

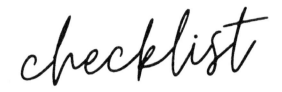

checklist

Setting up a Support System

- [ ] Identify family, friends and neighbors you can rely on for help

- [ ] Tell them about your surgery

- [ ] Let them know how they can help you prepare for surgery and the recovery

- [ ] Find support groups online or in your community

- [ ] Assign them tasks others can't help you with

- [ ] Stay in touch with your support team

- [ ] Thank your support team with words of appreciation and your actions

I'd love to hear from you!

Many women are still misinformed about a hysterectomy and base their decisions on fear, myths and misconceptions. Others are struggling with post-hysterectomy symptoms and need help navigating these issues.

Please consider leaving a review on Amazon to spread the word and help more women benefit from this resource so they can be inspired, too.

To leave a review, open the camera on your phone and scan the QR code below or use the link in your Amazon order to launch the review page.

It only takes 60 seconds.

Chapter 6

WHAT TO EXPECT ON SURGERY DAY

"Beyond drama and chaos, beyond anxiety and fear, lies a zone of endless peace and love. Let's all take a very deep breath, slow down for just a moment and remember this. That alone will open the door..."

MARIANNE WILLIAMSON

I was petrified on the day of surgery, with scary thoughts haunting me, "What if I don't make it? What if the surgery is unsuccessful?" So, I prayed, and in the end, God gave me peace.

I told myself that if I didn't survive, I would end up in His loving arms, and He would take care of my loved ones. If I survived, that was His will, too.

Thankfully, the surgery was successful, and the nurses were amazing.

Knowing what to expect can put your mind at ease. These days, most of us only go somewhere *after* reading online reviews about it and looking at photos of the place.

I don't even visit a new restaurant without checking their menu first and managing my expectations. So, how can you go for a life-changing event, a hysterectomy, without learning what will happen each step of the way?

Keep reading to get a vivid picture of everything you can expect on the day of surgery — before, during and after the operation.

Although the procedure is generally the same, there may be differences in treatment, hospital protocols and processes, based on your surgeon's preferences.

As such, don't expect everything to go exactly as mentioned in this chapter.

Instead, speak with your surgeon directly if you need specifics about your hospital stay, patient rights, surgical technique or medications.

RIGHT BEFORE THE SURGERY

You'll book into the hospital a few hours before the operation, but your doctor will advise you on how early to arrive. You can check in at the registration desk or go to the ward floor. The nurses will be expecting you and may even have a room ready when you get there.

The first thing you'll do is **fill out a bunch of forms**. These may include:

- A personal information form
- A power of attorney form
- Insurance information
- A consent form, allowing the staff to take life-saving measures if needed
- A form to conduct tests and insert tubes and monitoring devices during your stay

The nurses will leave you to **settle in your room** and acclimate with the ward. You can use this time to put your things away or make the room feel homey.

You'll have a **pre-op consultation** with the ward nurse, surgeon and anesthesiologist.

You'll share your medical history, any medications and prescriptions you're taking, habits (smoking, alcohol use, etc.), and if you've had any negative experiences with anesthesia or previous surgeries. Your doctor may also take this time to review procedural details with you and answer any lingering questions.

They may confirm that you've followed their instructions for pre-op preparation, such as drinking the bowel cleansing fluid and bathing with antiseptic soap.

You'll sign consent forms, permitting the team to perform the surgery and administer all necessary medications during the procedure.

You may be asked to choose your **menu preferences** for the next day. Since you've been restricted to light meals and liquids, you might be tempted to request a lot.

Try not to go overboard, as you may not have an appetite following surgery.

You may undergo a few necessary tests as well. These may include a blood test, chest X-ray and an electrocardiogram to check your heart.

If there are a few hours before the procedure, you'll have **some time to rest.** Otherwise, you'll receive pre-op medications, such as a mild tranquilizer, antibiotics and fluids.

You'll **change into a backless surgical gown and hat.** This is for hygiene and will give surgeons proper access to the surgical site.

You'll say goodbye to your friends and family around this time. Nurses generally don't allow many outsiders near you once you're in the sterilized outfit and given the pre-op medications.

In some hospitals, you can change your clothes and get the medications in your hospital room. In others, there's a separate area for all pre-op patients where nurses can better monitor your vitals and ensure a sterilized environment.

DURING SURGERY

When the operating room (OR) is ready, nurses will wheel you to surgery on a bed or wheelchair. The OR might feel robotic and foreign, with many stainless-steel tools and machines and an antiseptic smell.

After entering the OR, you'll move to the operating table. The surgical nurse will introduce themselves to you and inform you of the next step, which is anesthesia.

The entire surgery takes one to three hours.

It'll begin with anesthesia. If you're undergoing general anesthesia, the doctor will place a breathing tube inside your mouth or a mask over your mouth and nose. Then, they may ask you to count backward, and you'll soon lose consciousness.

The staff will insert a urinary catheter in you because you can't control that reflex under anesthesia. They'll clean the surgical area as well.

The following steps will depend on the type of hysterectomy you are having.

ABDOMINAL HYSTERECTOMY

Surgeons will make a 6–8-inch incision vertically or horizontally (along the bikini line in your abdomen). They'll detach the blood vessels and structures supporting the uterus and remove the uterus or fallopian tubes through the incision. They'll then close the incision with staples, sutures or surgical adhesive.

Anesthesiologists and respiratory therapists will monitor your vitals and breathing.

You'll be covered in a sterilized sheet with only the surgical area exposed. Once the procedure ends, you'll be gradually weaned off the anesthesia.

LAPAROSCOPIC HYSTERECTOMY

The surgeons will make 3-6 small incisions in your belly and insert surgical instruments and a camera. [38,39]

They'll use these tools to detach the blood vessels, then cut the structures and organs they need to take out into small pieces and remove them.

Some techniques remove the pieces through the surgical instruments in the belly, while others remove them through the vagina. In the case of the vaginal route, your legs will be placed in stirrups.

At the end of the surgery, the small incisions will be closed with sutures or surgical adhesive, and the anesthesia will be slowly removed from your system.

VAGINAL HYSTERECTOMY

In this procedure, your legs will be in stirrups for better access. Surgeons will make a small incision in the upper part of the vagina and insert sterile instruments there. They'll detach the uterus from blood vessels and supporting structures and remove it in pieces. You can be under general anesthesia or epidural.

During general anesthesia, you'll be unconscious and the pain dampened. In the case of an epidural, you'll be awake but won't feel anything. The surgical staff will place a curtain over your belly, so you won't see what's happening below.

IMMEDIATELY AFTER SURGERY

After surgery, you'll be moved to a recovery area, where your vital signs will be closely monitored. The breathing tube will be removed if your breathing is normal.

Nurses and surgeons will monitor you for pain and medicate you as needed. When you are stable, you'll be moved from the recovery area to your hospital room, where you'll be monitored for a day or two.

At this time, you can meet family and friends and have one or two people stay with you in the room.

Here are some things you can expect once you are awake:

- Pain over the surgical site

- A bandage on your belly or vagina

- A tube coming out of the surgical site (mostly in an abdominal hysterectomy; removed in 1-2 days)

- IV in your arm or hand

- A urine catheter (removed 24 hours post-surgery)

- A pad or gauze near your vagina to absorb blood

You may be in a lot of pain, feel **tired and groggy,** and like you need to use the bathroom. You may also have a horrible **sore throat** from having tubes in your throat, but it should resolve within two days. You can request a throat lozenge for relief.

If you had a total or radical hysterectomy, where both ovaries were removed, you'll go into menopause right away. You may experience a sense of loss from no longer having a uterus or being able to have children. These feelings are normal.

The hospital staff will check on you regularly and give you painkillers to relieve the discomfort.

You'll be **encouraged to walk around** soon after the procedure to increase blood circulation, prevent clots and alleviate gas or constipation. In addition, a physical therapist may help you move during your stay.

Although you may be relieved that the procedure is over, you may not feel the positive effects immediately or until the surgical pain dissipates.

You may also have **little to no appetite,** which will improve over time. It may hurt to laugh, sneeze and cough because it puts pressure on your wounds.

While you're still at the hospital, ask the doctor and staff any remaining questions you may have. Jot down some notes you can reference later in case you forget. It's easy to feel disoriented or confused after surgery.

Here are some questions you may have:

- How should I nurse my incisions? What type of bandages can I use?
- When can I shower and start taking regular baths?
- How can I reduce constipation?
- Can I bend down or make my bed?
- What are my lifting restrictions?

- Can I go up and down the stairs?

- How and when can I wean off the medication?

Having a family member or friend with you is helpful while the doctor answers these questions. Including those who'll be your primary caretakers is even better. It'll save you from having to relay the information to them later. You can also compare notes if you misinterpret any instructions.

GOOD TO KNOW

After surgery, you may be surprised you're still in tremendous pain. Many women opt for a hysterectomy to fix this discomfort and treat severe health problems. So, naturally, you may expect the agony to end as soon as you remove the organs causing the pain. But that's not always the case.

The procedure itself is painful. In time, the discomfort will diminish and eventually go away.

In the meantime, you may need medications to manage the pain. You'll want to take the meds before the pain becomes unbearable, so you can stay ahead of it.

You may **sleep a lot** and feel **constipated and gassy**. These are typical. Drinking water will help with constipation. Taking short walks or moving around can push out some of the trapped gas. You can also tackle this with proper diet and nutrition.

Additionally, if you're battling constipation, you can ask

your doctor to prescribe a stool softener to help with bowel movements while you're home.

You may also experience **nausea** from the anesthesia. Most women feel nauseous for 3-4 days, but you may feel ill for a couple of weeks.

You may also have **vaginal discharge** for up to 8 weeks. The discharge may be bloody, but should lighten up. Notify your doctor if it doesn't or is accompanied by intense pain.

Here are some ways to make your hospital stay more comfortable:

- Bring pillows, soft toys or a blanket for comfort.

- Bring your toiletries and soft slippers.

- Bring distractions to take your mind off the pain and hospital environment.

- Listen to the doctors and nurses. They care for patients daily and know what might help.

- Don't feel bad about resting. Your loved ones are there to assist you. Let them care for you and the logistics while you focus on healing.

- If possible, have someone jot down how to care for your wounds as a refresher for when you're home.

- Have a loved one with you throughout the stay to notice changes in your pain levels and bleeding and to inform the nurses right away.

- Have someone advocate on your behalf. It'll take a load off your shoulders.

- Put a loved one in charge of updating your family and friends so you won't have to.

- Limit visitors so you can rest.

Having the right doctor, hospital and team makes a world of difference.

Let me introduce you to Laura Langolf. She chose a laparoscopic hysterectomy so she could have the quickest recovery. Her hospital honored her wishes throughout her stay, providing an "excellent" experience — her words.

I can imagine that this experience positively influenced her post-op recovery as well.[40]

Similarly, Amy Schemur filmed a short video from her hospital bed showing how well the staff and her husband cared for her. She had a great hospital stay as well.[41]

Talia had a good experience at the hospital after her hysterectomy. She came prepared and communicated her needs and preferences to the doctor in advance.[42]

Let's review what you can expect on the day of surgery:

- You'll check in at the hospital a few hours before surgery, fill out forms and hand your list of medications to the nurse.

- You'll have a pre-op consultation and sign a consent form for surgery.

- You'll change into a surgical gown and move to the pre-op area.

- The nurses will wheel you into the operating room and move you to the operating table.

- You'll undergo anesthesia and a urinary catheter will be inserted.

- Depending on the type of surgery, you'll get incisions on your belly or vagina.

- After surgery, you'll be moved to a recovery area while the anesthesia wears off.

- You can meet your loved ones once you're back in your room after gaining consciousness.

- You may experience pain at the surgical site. A tube may come out of the incisions, and you will have an IV in your arm.

- After the procedure, you may feel tired, dizzy, constipated, gassy, pain and have a sore throat.

- You should ask your doctor important questions about caring for your incisions and overall health before leaving the hospital.

Next, we'll discuss what to expect once you're released.

Chapter 7

POST-OP NEED-TO-KNOWS

"It's always hard to deal with injuries mentally, but I like to think about it as a new beginning. I can't change what happened, so the focus needs to go toward healing and coming back stronger than before."

CARLI LLOYD

Healing doesn't have a clock. How fast your body heals depends on the type of hysterectomy and your overall health condition. For example, it can take 6 to 8 weeks for large incisions to heal from an abdominal hysterectomy, but 4 to 6 weeks if you had laparoscopic surgery.

Other factors may also extend your recovery period, such as stress, an unsupportive environment, pre-existing medical conditions and some medications.

It's tempting to want to rush the process, but unfortunately, this can land you back in surgery. That's why it's important to listen to your body and let it mend at its own pace. Your patience will pay off in the long run.

Here are some essentials to know for proper recovery as you adjust to life back home.

PHASES OF WOUND HEALING

Blood clotting is the first step of wound healing. It happens almost immediately after your incisions are closed.

Inflammation is the next phase and can last up to a week post-surgery. During this time, your body kills bacteria, removes debris and brings oxygen, nutrients and white blood cells to the surgical site. You may experience some pain, swelling and a slight redness.

Here, you'll want to watch out for infection. The telltale signs of an infection are:

- Oozing wound
- Smelly discharge from the incision area
- Redness, pain and swelling persist after a week
- The pain gets worse
- The area feels hot
- Fever
- Increased vaginal bleeding

Next, is the **rebuilding phase,** which lasts 4-30 days after the procedure.

Your body repairs the damaged area, stitching together separated muscles, tissues and skin layers. The area under the incision line thickens with new collagen and may feel like a semi-hard mass as scar tissue forms.

The firmness should soften and flatten in about 2 to 3 weeks after surgery.

The final and longest phase is **remodeling,** lasting 21 days to 2 years after surgery.

During this time, collagen production continues. The wound slowly shrinks, and new fibers reorganize as they blend with healthy neighboring skin. Over time, your scar will mature and change color.[43]

DISCHARGE DAY

Your release day may vary from **1-2 days** after surgery (if you had a laparoscopic or vaginal hysterectomy) to **4-5 days** afterward (for an open abdominal procedure).

On the other hand, if the hysterectomy was due to cancer, your stay may be extended, regardless of the approach. You may also require cancer-related treatments (chemotherapy or radiotherapy) or need to wait for test results. Your oncologist will clarify this beforehand.

The staff may use a wheelchair to transport you to your car. During the transfer, your insides may feel like they're falling apart.

Once in the car, place a soft pillow between your stomach and the seat belt. This will make it less painful to fasten the seat belt and provide much-needed cushioning.

I felt every bump on the road and each time the car started and stopped, although my daughter drove carefully. This may be true for you, too, so don't be afraid to take pain meds for the trip.

Brace yourself for the mixed emotions you may feel as you leave the care of professionals and return home, where you'll primarily care for yourself.

Have someone pick up your prescriptions if that still needs to happen. If your loved ones are available, share your notes with them so they can properly dress your wounds or administer medication.

ADJUSTING AT HOME

You may **sleep a lot** in the first week. This is good for you, so don't fight it. You may also **feel constipated** for several days for various reasons:

- Narcotic pain relievers, such as opioids, slow down the digestive system.

- Anesthesia can affect bowel function. It paralyzes your intestines and stops the movement of stool while it's in your system.

- Changes in diet (such as not eating or drinking before surgery or being put on a restrictive diet afterward) can affect digestion. Less fluid results in hard, dry and immobile stools.

- Inactivity may contribute to constipation.

Thankfully, you can increase your water intake to alleviate constipation. Eating high-fiber foods, such as nuts, carrots, whole grains, berries and apples with their skin, can help.

Your doctor may also prescribe a stool softener. Take the laxative as directed in the days following surgery, then ease off over time.

It's typical not to have a **bowel movement** for the first few days, but if you're experiencing issues after 5 days, contact your doctor.

After surgery, you may also develop occasional **abdominal cramps, gas and bloating.** This temporary pain happens as gas builds up in the intestines.

You can try nonprescription medications (e.g., simethicone [sample brand name: Gas-X]) to relieve the gas and bloating.

Other ways to reduce gas and cramping include:

- Eliminating gassy foods and drinks
- Walking
- Using a heating pad

Call your surgeon if the pain or bloating is severe or does not resolve after a week. They can prescribe medication or order tests to diagnose the problem.

You may continue to experience **nausea** for up to 10 weeks after surgery. The average timeline for nausea is 7 weeks if you had a vaginal hysterectomy and 9 weeks if you had a total hysterectomy.[44]

Note: These numbers don't apply to everyone, so only use them as a guide.

Moreover, you may continue **bleeding** for up to 8 weeks after surgery. If your bleeding is heavier than a pink discharge or increases over time, contact your doctor to confirm it's not serious.

If you have laparoscopic surgery, you may experience **shoulder pain** from the gas used to expand your abdomen during the operation. The shoulder pain may last a few days, but symptoms will generally improve when sitting or standing.

Over-the-counter pain relievers, heat therapy and gentle stretching exercises may alleviate this pain.

You may also find it challenging to **sit up in bed** because of your sutures. Sitting upright can add pressure to your back and stomach. If you must sit, try reclining, but shift your position every one to two hours so you're not in the same spot for an extended time.

MANAGING YOUR PAIN LEVELS

Not everyone needs medication to manage their pain. However, if you need painkillers, don't feel guilty. Excessive pain can slow down your healing and impact your mood and sleep quality.

When it comes to pain management, here are some tips to keep in mind:

- To stay ahead of the pain, **take the medicine** as prescribed *before* you need it, then work with your doctor to eventually reduce and wean off it.

- Waiting too long to take medications can make the pain unbearable or last longer.

- Read the medicine's label for dosage, timing, possible side effects and precautions, then follow the instructions religiously.

- Taking painkillers more frequently or at a higher dose than recommended is unsafe and may cause accidental overdose or harm.

It's easy to lose track of time when taking medicine. I jotted down each time I took my meds so I wouldn't take them sooner than required or forget about them.

Below are some reminder apps you can try:

- Medisafe
- MyTherapy
- Pill Reminder – All in One
- Express Scripts
- EveryDose

Many painkillers are available over the counter, and you can get the rest by prescription. These can either be non-opioid (non-narcotic) or opioid (narcotic).

Because opioid medications are strong and addictive, they're only available through prescription. However, non-opioid options are safer, less powerful and non-addictive, so don't require a prescription.

Non-opioid pain medications include acetaminophen (sample brand name: Tylenol) and ibuprofen (sample brand names: Advil, Motrin). Opioid pain medications include tramadol, oxycodone, hydrocodone and hydromorphone.

Your doctor may prescribe pain medications combining acetaminophen (non-opioid) with an opioid (containing acetaminophen) and one of the following: [45]

- oxycodone (Percocet)
- codeine (Tylenol 3)
- Hydrocodone (Vicodin)

Check with them for usage and which medications you can take together. It's important not to drink alcohol or take other meds containing acetaminophen concurrently with your opioid medication if it also contains acetaminophen, as acetaminophen may cause liver damage when taken in excess. [45]

Wear **loose, comfortable clothing and undergarments** that promote healing, rather than garments that pull at your incisions. I found knitted underwear to work best.

Try to avoid **uncomfortable positions or activities,** such as bending forward and sitting in low chairs. Instead, support your abdomen with a folded blanket or pillow or use a belly wrap. [45]

Applying this reinforcement can offer psychological and physical support while changing positions.

Place a **hot water bottle or heating pad** on your stomach for 15-20 minutes to relieve cramping or nausea. Keep the heat low and put a towel or cloth in between to prevent burns.

Treat **constipation and gas** with medication and diet for better sleep and comfort.

REST

Rest is essential for optimal recovery. Sleep enhances your body's ability to repair and stimulates tissue growth so you can heal faster.

Stay in bed as much as possible during the first 2 weeks. You can do gentle exercises to keep the blood flowing from the comfort of your bed.

Resting at the hospital isn't ideal, and you may have short-term insomnia from the anesthesia. The bright lights, beeping machines, constant interruptions, pain, discomfort and new location also contribute to insomnia.

You may continue to experience insomnia once you're home because of the pain, discomfort, nausea, bloating and side effects of medication. To reduce insomnia for better rest:

- Manage your anxiety

- Take pain medication on time

- Create a dark, comfortable environment. (Use earplugs and an eye mask and control the room's temperature.)

Adjusting to your new sleeping position can be difficult, especially if you're a stomach sleeper. Lying on your stomach is discouraged for the first few weeks after a hysterectomy. It can take 2 to 6 weeks to return to regular sleep patterns.

Here's a breakdown of your options by surgery type.

If you had a robotic or abdominal procedure, you should avoid sleeping on your stomach or side, as it puts pressure on the incisions. Sleeping on your back in a slightly elevated position is preferred.

When sleeping on your back, place a pillow underneath your knees to alleviate back pain.

If you had a laparoscopic surgery, you should not sleep on your stomach or the side with incisions. However, you can sleep on your back or the alternate side without incisions.

Sleeping sideways may alleviate gas pain. When sleeping on your side, place one pillow between your legs and the other against your body for support. This will keep the pelvis from rolling and support your lower abdomen.

FOOD AND NUTRITION

Since you won't move much after surgery, eat **small meals** and only what you can tolerate, then stop when you're satisfied.

Make a note of the foods you're eating and how they make you feel. Also, **watch your calories** if weight gain is a concern. At the same time, don't eat too little to avoid weight gain. Macros and calorie tracking can help you stay ahead of excess weight while you recuperate.

Eat a **well-balanced diet** with lots of fiber and drink plenty of water to alleviate constipation.

An **anti-inflammatory diet** may reduce pain. These include fruits and vegetables, foods containing omega-3 fatty acids, whole grains, lean protein, healthy fats and spices.

Supplement your diet with extra protein, vitamin C, vitamin D, zinc, probiotics, collagen, curcumin and such. These boost immunity and promote wound healing and muscle growth.

WOUND CARE

When it comes to wound care, following your doctor's advice is crucial. Taking care of your incisions reduces scarring and the risk of an infection.

Try not to submerge your cuts in water or take a bath. Wait at least 24 hours after surgery before showering. If you take a shower, dry the area with a clean towel as soon as you can.

Your **staples and some stitches** are removed before you leave the hospital. If you have any remaining stitches that don't dissolve on their own, they can be removed at your surgeon's office 5-7 days post-surgery.

Stitches under your skin or within the vagina will dissolve in a few weeks. You may notice parts of the stitching on your undergarments as they come out.

If the surgeon uses **surgical glue** to close your wound, try not to soak or remove the glue for the first week or until the cut has healed. Instead, gently pat the area dry. If the glue doesn't peel off after 5-10 days, use an ointment to carefully remove it.

If you have **adhesive bandages,** these will come off on

their own in about 2 weeks. If they don't, wash your hands thoroughly, then soak the bandages in warm water. Once the bandages loosen, gently peel them off in the direction of hair growth. Repeat the process until they're all removed.

Wash the area around the wound with mild soap and water, then pat it dry and place a fresh dressing on the wound.

It's important to change your dressing every day to prevent infection. Always wash your hands beforehand, cleaning the skin surrounding your incisions with mild soap or saline solution and water, but avoid using alcohol, hydrogen peroxide, lotion, creams, iodine or antibacterial chemicals on the area.

Your surgeon may want you to cover the wound or leave it open, but they'll confirm.

If you're unsure whether you have an infection, revisit the warning signs at the beginning of this chapter and contact your doctor if anything looks or feels out of place.

Maintaining a healthy diet, not smoking and massaging the scar can **enhance recovery.** Some women find infrared lamp therapy beneficial, but there's insufficient evidence that it speeds up healing.[46]

TAKING CARE OF YOUR MENTAL HEALTH

Support a good mindset during recovery. Here are some recommendations:

- **Journal** how you're feeling.

- **Shower** and change your pajamas.

- Open the curtains and windows. **Sunlight** is a mood booster.

- **Freshen your room** or ask someone to help.

- Sprinkle pleasant **aromatherapy oils** like lavender and bergamot in the room.

- Have fresh **flowers** delivered.

- Surround yourself with **positive people.**

- Take a **short walk** or sit in your sunroom or garden for fresh air.

- Spend time with loved ones.

- Engage in **light-hearted entertainment,** such as listening to music or reading a book.

- Do some **physical activity** every day. You can try exercises in bed if that's where you spend most of your time.

GENERAL RECOMMENDATIONS FOR RECOVERY

LIFTING

Try not to lift anything heavier than 10 pounds for the first six weeks. Also, avoid heavy housework and other strenuous activities. Lifting the wrong way can put too much pressure on your wound and tear the incisions.

BENDING

Limit forward-bending movements, such as making your bed, doing laundry and vacuuming. Frequent bending while your wound is fresh may cause a prolapse or an incisional hernia, where a lump or bulge develops at the surgical site.

A post-hysterectomy prolapse can happen at any time, as shown in this 2014 report from the Journal of The Society of Laparoscopic & Robotic Surgeons:

> *"The cumulative risk is described as 1% three years after hysterectomy and up to 15% fifteen years later."*[47]

Similarly, an incisional hernia may not present until three months or even a year post-surgery, but can occur at any time.

STAIRS

If you use steps, take them one at a time after the procedure. Then, as you build up your strength, take the stairs as much as you can tolerate over the following weeks.

DRIVING

Do not drive for at least two weeks until you can safely start and stop the vehicle and wear a seatbelt without pain.

Opioids, anesthesia and painkillers may compromise your reaction time, decision-making and focus, so it's best not to drive until you've fully weaned off the medication.

SEXUAL ACTIVITIES

You should ideally wait 4-6 weeks to resume penetrative sexual activity so your incisions have time to heal and the vaginal discharge stops. Your doctor may give you the green light sooner.

Engaging in penetrative sex too early may reopen your wound, cause bleeding or trigger an infection.

WEIGHT MANAGEMENT

Weight can creep up fast after a hysterectomy. Some reasons why this happens include:

- Hormonal change
- More time in bed
- Lack of exercise
- Diet and nutrition

To stay ahead of it, plan for weight management before the procedure. This can be difficult, particularly if you are physically and mentally exhausted or battling other health-related issues.

Here are a few tips:

- Focus on maintaining nutrition while cutting extra sugar and carbs

- Drink plenty of water

- Get adequate sleep

- Manage stress through positive affirmations or therapy

- Exercise

- Invite friends or family to help if needed

- Journal to track daily habits and see where you can include more healthy activities

PHYSICAL ACTIVITY AND EXERCISE

Stay active after surgery, but avoid strenuous activities for the first six weeks. Increase the activity's duration or intensity when you're ready for it, but don't force it if anything hurts.

Start with light exercises, such as **walking.** It gets the bowels moving and reduces the risk of blood clots.

With your doctor's approval, try **low-impact exercises** like light stretching, yoga or Kegels a few times a day. You can also swim, but only after your wounds have closed and the vaginal bleeding and discharge have stopped.

Refrain from high-impact exercises until your physician gives you the go-ahead, roughly 6-8 weeks after the hysterectomy.

WHEN TO CONTACT YOUR DOCTOR

Take note of what's normal and abnormal as you heal. This may include any differences with your incisions, constipation, pain, bloating, gas, energy levels and vaginal discharge. If anything is out of the ordinary, contact your doctor for help.

Also, reach out if any new symptoms emerge, such as chest pain, fever or redness around the wound.

Let's review the post-op need-to-knows:

- Your **wound heals** in phases. The blood clots first, then there's swelling and redness. The wound hardens and finally blends in with your skin.

- You're typically **discharged** within 1 to 2 days for a vaginal hysterectomy and 4 to 5 days for an abdominal procedure.

- Grab a pillow for the ride home.

- **Sleep** as much as you need in the initial days for improved recovery.

- Drink plenty of **water** and eat a high-fiber diet to avoid constipation.

- You may experience **nausea, bleeding and shoulder pain** in the days following surgery.

- Take **medications** before the pain gets unbearable.

- Rushing your recovery may cause more damage.

- To promote healing, wear loose, comfortable **clothing** and avoid uncomfortable positions.

- Eat **small meals** and track your calories, but keep a well-balanced and nutritious diet.

- Your doctor will **remove staples** and certain types of stitches before you leave the hospital or in their office days after surgery. Internal stitches will dissolve on their own.

- **Wash your hands** before tending to your wounds and **change your dressings daily** to prevent infection.

- To improve your **mental** well-being, practice gratitude, spend time with your loved ones and in nature, and engage in light-hearted entertainment.

- Don't **lift** anything heavier than 10 pounds for the first six weeks. Limit **bending down.**

- Avoid **driving** for at least two weeks and when you're no longer taking meds.

- If you use **steps**, take them one at a time.

- Wait 4-6 weeks to resume **penetrative sexual activities**.

- Manage your **weight** through diet and exercise.

You are now covered for your recovery time at home.

Sometimes, things don't go as planned or something just doesn't feel right. We'll discuss what you can do about post-operative problems that may arise, so you're prepared.

In the meantime, here's a healthy lifestyle, eating and exercise plan you can try after surgery.

POST-OP HEALTHY LIFESTYLE EXERCISE PLAN	
Exercise Type	*Exercise Options* *(Slowly increase duration over time.)*
Aerobic exercise	• Walking • Stationary bike/cycling
Stretching and mobility	• Light yoga • Gentle stretching
Pelvic floor muscle exercises	• Kegels • Pelvic tilts

POST-OP HEALTHY LIFESTYLE FOOD PLAN	
Food Type	*Food Options*
Try adding colorful foods to your plate for each meal. **(*These options are some of the best sources of antioxidants, so try to include them.*)**	• *Red:* Cranberries, red grapes, peaches, raspberries, strawberries, red currants, figs, cherries • *Orange:* Oranges, pumpkin, carrots, apricots, mangoes, sweet potatoes, butternut squash, kabocha squash • *Yellow:* Lemons, banana, sweetcorn, kūmara, swede, yellow/orange bell peppers (capsicums), carrots, yams and the pumpkin group • *Deep Green:* Salad greens, kale and spinach, broccoli, bok choy and mustard
Try to consume *high-fiber meals* daily	• Oatmeal, brown rice, whole wheat pasta and cereals • Black, red and kidney beans
Try to include *lean protein sources* with every meal	• Skinless chicken • Fatty fish like salmon (with omega-3 fats) • Vegetable protein
Try increasing your *calcium intake* to counter the lack of estrogen	• Low-fat dairy (8oz, 4 servings) • Hard cheese • Yogurt • Fortified products like orange juice, canned salmon, broccoli and legumes

Chapter 8

DEALING WITH DILEMMAS

While post-op problems may happen, it helps to know there are possible solutions if they do.

Most post-op complications can be monitored and treated while you're at the hospital. However, once you're at home, it's vital to take note of any issues, even if they're not serious.

Since you're no longer under the watchful eye of the hospital team, your best line of defense begins with you.

Here are 7 common post-op dilemmas you may encounter:

1. Early menopause or surgical menopause

2. Infection

3. Blood clots

4. Pain

5. Weight gain

6. Pelvic floor muscle weakness and urinary leakage

7. Organ shift or prolapse

Depending on your surgery, you may not experience any of these issues, or you may experience one or multiple issues. Knowing the warning signs is the first step in achieving success.

EARLY MENOPAUSE OR SURGICAL MENOPAUSE

If your ovaries are removed during the hysterectomy, you'll immediately enter menopause.

Removal or damage to the ovaries results in a rapid drop in estrogen. This sudden change in hormone levels may result in the following exaggerated menopausal symptoms:

- Hot flashes
- Vaginal dryness and decreased libido
- Mood swings
- Difficulty sleeping
- Weight gain
- Hair loss or thinning hair
- Night sweats
- Dry skin, jowls and slack skin
- Urinary incontinence
- Rapid heartbeat

On the other hand, if your ovaries are retained, you may still experience early menopause within a few years. Research shows that after a hysterectomy, the ovaries fail quicker than if you don't have the procedure.[47]

TREATMENT

Menopause and early menopause are irreversible, but you can manage the symptoms through lifestyle changes or Hormone Replacement Therapy.

Lifestyle changes include:

- **Diet:** Limit caffeine and alcohol. Add fruits, vegetables and sources of calcium, such as milk, yogurt and kale, to your diet.

- **Exercise:** Regular exercise reduces weight gain, balances your mood and increases energy. Resistance training or weight-bearing activities also strengthen the bones.

- **Mood management/CBT:** Spending time with loved ones, enjoying nature, volunteering, praying and maintaining a good sleep routine improves mood. You may also find cognitive behavioral therapy (CBT) with a certified psychologist beneficial.

- **Smoking.** If you smoke or you stopped smoking temporarily, try to kick the habit permanently. Replace smoking with healthier habits you enjoy, such as calling a friend, journaling or completing a jigsaw puzzle.

- **Manage hot flashes and night sweats** by limiting spicy foods, wearing loose clothing, taking cold showers, and installing a fan or an air conditioner in your room.

Some women find Hormone Replacement Therapy (HRT) helpful. HRT comes in different forms, including:

- Oral tablets
- Skin patches

- An implant inside the body. This is placed under anesthesia.

- Estrogen gel you can rub on your skin.

- Estrogen sprays you can apply to your skin.

- Ovestin Pessaries you can insert in the vagina.

- Vaginal creams

HRT has several side effects, however. You may experience nausea, leg cramps, breast changes and depression. HRT also increases the risk of breast cancer and blood clots.

Hormone Replacement Therapy may be unsuitable if you have cancer or precancerous cells. I chose not to try HRT, but that's not to say you shouldn't.

INFECTION

About 10% of women develop an infection after a hysterectomy. Three percent develop a surgical site infection even if they receive antibiotics before surgery.[48]

Women with an *abdominal* hysterectomy are more likely to develop infections than those with a *vaginal* hysterectomy. On rare occasions, the infection will form an abscess (a collection of bacteria and pus) and may need to be drained. Symptoms of a post-op infection may include:

- Fever

- Chills

- Cold sweats

- Shortness of breath

- Pus oozing from the surgical site

- Pain, redness and heat around the wound site

- Burning or pain with urination (especially if there's a urinary tract infection)

- Nausea or vomiting

TREATMENT

It's important to **see your doctor** if you develop a post-op infection. They may prescribe antibiotics to manage it. Take the **medication** for at least a week. The length of time may vary, depending on the severity or type of infection.

You also may need surgery (wound exploration and debridement) to treat the infection. Here, your doctor will examine the surgical site, determine how far the infection has spread, and remove as much infected tissue as possible.

Infections are not to be taken lightly. They can start superficially in the skin, then move to the deeper layers of muscles and organs if they're not treated promptly.

TIPS FOR AVOIDING AN INFECTION

Post-op antibiotics are excellent for avoiding infection. To reduce the likelihood of an infection:

- Thoroughly follow your doctor's instructions for

cleaning and dressing your wound.

- Keep your hands clean and use antibacterial soap whenever you wash your hands.

- Don't leave your wound open in an unsanitary or highly-polluted environment.

- Avoid tobacco, alcohol and foods that weaken your immune system.

- Don't apply any unprescribed ointment to the wound while it is fresh.

Keep a close eye on your incisions for the first two weeks. Your surgeon will likely check the surgical area at post-op visits and tell you when it's safe to stop dressing the wound and ease up on sanitary precautions.

BLOOD CLOTS

Blood clots after surgery (venous thromboembolism) affect about 1% of women after a hysterectomy.[49] You may develop a blood clot 2-10 days after surgery, but your odds remain high for up to 3 months.

These clots can travel inside your body and deposit in sensitive areas, such as your heart or lungs. As such, following the doctor's orders is key.

Blood clots may present with the following symptoms:

- Throbbing or cramping pain, swelling, redness, and

warmth in a leg or arm

- Sudden breathlessness, light-headedness

- Sharp chest pain and a cough

To reduce the risk of blood clot, move your arms and legs in bed or walk as much as possible. Low-intensity exercises in bed also keep the blood flowing.

TREATMENT

Because clots can be life-threatening, you may need **immediate medical assistance** if you notice any of the symptoms mentioned earlier. Additionally, your doctor may prescribe a blood thinner to treat or prevent clots post-surgery.

PAIN

It's normal to experience post-surgery pain at the wound site or from gas or constipation. However, you may experience other types of pain as well. For example:

- Your **throat** may hurt because of anesthesia, and you may have trouble swallowing and eating for a few days.

- You may have occasional **back pain** due to spinal anesthesia. Long-term back pain may be due to the negative impact on pelvic areas and organs.

- **Scar tissue** can cause pain months after the procedure. It may exaggerate during your menstrual cycle (if your ovaries weren't removed).

- Nerve endings send signals of pain, touch and pressure to the brain. Sometimes, the reproductive organs send pain signals when they shouldn't. This shooting or **neuropathic pain** can be due to a nerve injury and may present as tingling, numbness, muscle weakness or burning.

Not all pain is bad, however. Some are mild, temporary and not serious. You can assess and monitor your pain level using various scales, such as:

- **Numeric rating scales (NRS).** These rate your pain level from 0 to 10, with 10 indicating the most severe.

- **Visual analog scale (VAS).** You pick a spot on the line (with 0 written on one end and 10 on the other) based on how much pain you're in.

- **Categorical scale**. There are emojis or images of faces in different colors on a chart. You pick the one that represents you best.

When to contact your doctor:

- If the pain **is unbearable** or becomes unmanageable.

- If the pain **persists or worsens.** (You'll generally experience less pain while doing everyday activities over time.)

- If you're experiencing **extreme pain or discomfort three months post-surgery.** In addition to seeing your physician, you may benefit from seeing a pain specialist to determine the root cause.

TREATMENT

Everyone deals with post-op pain differently. I was in excruciating pain for weeks following my hysterectomy, and it was difficult to taper off the medication. Thanks to my support system, who managed my meds, I was able to wean off the oxycodone successfully.

In my case, I slowly transitioned to a mixture of prescription and over-the-counter meds, then switched to over-the-counter meds (without any oxy), and eventually stopped the meds altogether.

One way to treat your pain is with medication. Some pain medications can be addictive or even dangerous when combined with other medications, however. (Refer to Chapter 7 for precautions to take.) Alternative treatment options are also available, such as physical therapy.

If a specific activity aggravates your pain, try stopping it for a while. Then, after a few days, carefully revisit the activity and see if the pain returns. Doing too much too soon can result in unnecessary pain, but easing into activities can alleviate it.

A physical therapist can help you modify activities and avoid painful postures and tasks. You can also try the following:

- Practice **gratitude** and **affirmations** to manage and reduce stress

- Muscle-strengthening **exercises**

- Heat, cold and **massage therapy** for temporary comfort from pain

WEIGHT GAIN

Menopause reduces your body's estrogen levels, triggering metabolic changes. Women tend to lose muscle mass, burn less calories and gain weight during this transition. Studies show that women gain an average of 1 pound per year, with 20% gaining 10 or more pounds.[50]

Because a hysterectomy may result in surgical menopause, you're more susceptible to weight gain afterward.

The ligaments in your pelvis may also weaken, causing the hips or butt to spread. Fat mainly accumulates around the waist after menopause, giving you a bigger belly.

Some women lose weight after surgery. However, others (including me) gain weight. I gained over 20 pounds within six months after my hysterectomy.

I was doing all the right things. I ate healthily and exercised regularly. My diet was primarily fruits and vegetables with some protein. I got at least 8 hours of rest, drank plenty of water, ate smaller meals throughout the day, and even ate my last meal a few hours before bedtime.

None of these things helped. Instead, my body seemed to have a mind of its own. I'd never had trouble losing weight before. But after the procedure, I felt like my metabolism was shot until I discovered the perfect cocktail of different steps that work together to keep my weight balanced.

You, too, may find it more challenging to lose weight after a hysterectomy and easier to pile on the pounds.

TIPS FOR MANAGING WEIGHT

Here are some things that worked for me that you can try as well:

- Track your food intake with an app. I journaled daily and noted my food intake and weight fluctuations.

- Move every day. Even 20-30 minutes of movement or exercise can make a difference.

- Watch your portion sizes and reduce them wisely.

- Aim to eat less sugar, processed foods and fats. Add more whole grains, lean meats, seeds, nuts, fish, poultry, eggs and complex carbs. (Revisit the "Food and nutrition" section in Chapter 7 or the "Two Months Before" section in Chapter 5.)

- Eat your last meal a few hours before bedtime to give your body time to digest it.

- Experiment with various diets, such as vegetarian or anti-inflammatory, to see which gives you the most energy and least significant weight gain.

- Incorporate intermittent fasting.

- Stand more than you sit once you're released to return

to your regular activities.

- Choose fats carefully. Moderately include healthy fats, such as those in nuts.

- Contact a nutritionist if you're stuck.

- Avoid mindless eating. Plan your snacks for the day and keep the rest out of sight.

- Don't ignore the power of a sound sleep routine.

By the way, if you're having trouble losing weight, you can grab my free gift for additional strategies at: https://www.hysterectomyfitness.com/discover

PELVIC FLOOR MUSCLE WEAKNESS AND URINARY LEAKAGE

In addition to triggering menopause, a hysterectomy can weaken your pelvic floor muscles when the uterus is removed, causing bladder control issues or uncontrollable urinary leakage (incontinence).

Other reasons for incontinence may include:

- Nerve damage to the bladder during surgery

- Damage to the muscles that control urine flow (urinary sphincter)

- Low estrogen levels may cause vaginal dryness if the ovaries are removed. Vaginal dryness may cause involuntary leakage or an urge to use the bathroom frequently.

You may not develop urinary incontinence until several years after a hysterectomy.

PubMed reports a 60% increase of developing urinary incontinence after a hysterectomy once you turn 60.[51]

Symptoms of a weak pelvic floor are:

- Leaking urine or incontinence. This may happen when you sneeze, cough, laugh or exercise.

- Reduced bowel control or fecal incontinence, where you fail to reach the bathroom in time.

- Pelvic organ prolapse

- Heaviness, fullness, pulling or aching in the vagina

- Difficulty urinating or emptying the bladder

- Constipation or straining during bowel movements

TREATMENT

Kegel exercises are one of the best ways to strengthen a weak pelvic floor. A pelvic floor physical therapist can train you how to perform these exercises and prescribe the most beneficial option for your problem.

Here are some other ways to manage urinary leakage or stress incontinence:

- Estrogen vaginal creams

- Wearing pads

- Medications (may include hormonal medications and oral pills)

- Bladder training through scheduling your bathroom visits and calculating fluid intake

- Urinary surgery to lift the bladder

- Vaginal pessaries, where you place silicon circular devices inside your vagina to help with incontinence

- Diet and lifestyle changes, such as reducing caffeine and losing weight

ORGAN SHIFT OR PROLAPSE

After a hysterectomy, your pelvic organs (the small intestine and reproductive organs) move to fill the space the uterus once occupied. This can put pressure on the muscles, tissues and ligaments.

It can also cause the organs to drop down in the pelvic cavity and bulge through the vagina, called a prolapse.

Nearly **40% of women** suffer from organ prolapse after a hysterectomy, but only **1.3 to 4.2 per 1000** women need surgical correction.[52,53]

The chances of developing prolapse are no different for abdominal, vaginal or laparoscopic hysterectomies.[54]

Symptoms of pelvic organ prolapse include:

- Pain in the pelvic area

- Feeling like you can't empty the bladder completely

- Urinary incontinence or urgency

- Difficulty inserting a tampon

- Bulging inside the vagina

- A portion of the vaginal vault protruding from the vagina (complete prolapse)

- Lower back pain

- Bladder and bowel infections

- Painful sexual intercourse

- Dragging pain in the abdomen

TREATMENT

Some surgical options for fixing organ prolapse include:

- **Sacrocolpopexy:** A piece of mesh attaches the vaginal vault to the tailbone to prevent organs from bulging.

- **Vaginal vault suspension:** The surgeon attaches the vagina to the pelvic ligaments to provide additional support.

- **Colpocleisis:** Sutures are applied to the vagina to close its opening and reduce the likelihood of another prolapse.

You can also try the following:

- **Medications**

- **Physical therapy:** Pelvic floor exercises are the go-to treatment for prolapse.

- **Pessaries:** These support the organs in the pelvis.

After learning about these post-op dilemmas, you may feel that a hysterectomy will result in many new problems. I was shaken up, too.

Thankfully, many of these issues are manageable with lifestyle modifications, diet, exercise, medication, and, in some cases, surgery.

Now, let's summarize what we've covered.

Here are the **key takeaways** regarding the specific post-op complications from this chapter:

- Be prepared for immediate **menopause** or early menopause after surgery.

- **Healthy lifestyle habits** like diet, exercise and mood management may reduce menopausal symptoms. While hormone replacement therapy is not for everyone, some women find it helpful.

- Watch out for **infection.** It can happen at the wound site or internally.

- The telltale signs of an infection are **fever, chills and pus** oozing from the surgical site. Contact your doctor immediately if you have an infection.

- You can manage post-op infections with medications and **good hygiene.**

- You may suffer from **blood clots** after surgery. Seek medical attention right away.

- After a hysterectomy, you may have a sore throat, back pain or pain from the scar tissue. Assess your pain and contact your doctor if it gets too bad or is persistent after three months.

- Having small meals throughout the day, tracking your food, consuming healthy fats, and exercising are some ways to manage post-op weight gain.

- **Pelvic floor muscle weakness** can cause urinary leakage, a feeling of heaviness in your vagina and fecal incontinence.

- Kegel exercises, urinary surgery and bladder training are ways to deal with urinary incontinence.

- **Pelvic organ prolapse** is a common post-op complication. You can opt for surgical repair, medication or physical therapy to treat it.

This life-changing surgery can take a toll on you mentally and physically. That's why we'll cover how to manage your mindset and physical well-being next.

Chapter 9

MANAGING YOUR MINDSET: DEALING WITH LOSS OF FEMININITY, FERTILITY AND POST-SURGICAL GRIEF

Researchers are unsure why some women experience increased anxiety and depression after surgery, although decreased estrogen can have a lot to do with that. There are many ways to support yourself during this time.

LEVINE, 2019

S tudies show that women sometimes feel a sense of loss after a hysterectomy, suffering from grief and mental issues no matter their age, even years after the procedure. This is because a hysterectomy doesn't just change you physically, but emotionally as well.

I know that hysterectomy is a sensitive subject and may be extremely painful.

You may have mixed emotions — depending on why you're undergoing surgery, if you can't keep your ovaries, or if you want to have kids.

I didn't expect to experience sadness following my surgery. I was shocked that I felt this way since I was able to retain my ovaries and already had a child.

Still, it was bittersweet. I couldn't believe that I missed having periods — the very thing that had caused me decades of pain and almost killed me. I share my battles, so you'll know that these feelings are normal.

Here are some cognitive and therapeutic tools that can help. They kept me positive and mentally healthy before and after surgery.

UNCOVERING YOUR CORE BELIEFS ABOUT GETTING A HYSTERECTOMY

Core beliefs are perceptions or assumptions we believe to be true. We use them as our North Star to guide our behaviors, decisions, feelings, actions and thoughts.

You may have core beliefs about getting a hysterectomy. Some of them may be positive or negative; others may be valid or invalid. In some cases, our core beliefs can keep us from making a scary, but important decision for our health.

Faulty beliefs may cause:

- Negative self-talk and anxiety
- Self-sabotage
- Missed opportunities

When I started my journey, my core beliefs about a hysterectomy were clouded; some positive and negative.

On one hand, I felt that a hysterectomy would not fully work and instead trigger other symptoms, such as weight gain and menopause, which I mentioned in earlier chapters. On the other hand, I was hopeful that it would eliminate my pain and gynecological issues.

In the end, it was a personal decision that only I could make, which is the same for you.

As you begin working through this process, identify your core beliefs about a hysterectomy. Dig deep. Ask yourself "why" and "how" you feel this way.

Use facts to weigh whether the belief is valid or invalid or if there are other options that'll work better for you. Aligning your beliefs with facts will improve your mental and physical health over time. If needed, revisit Chapters 1 and 3 on hysterectomy alternatives and decision-making.

Continue this cycle until you find the root of your worry or thoughts. This exercise may take time. Because core beliefs aren't developed overnight, reviewing their validity can be difficult.

UNDERSTANDING YOUR FEELINGS ARE NORMAL

For most women, opting for a hysterectomy is not entirely a *choice*. They're often in so much pain or physically beaten by this experience that they feel a hysterectomy is their last resort. As such, there's a sense of grief and helplessness.

Additionally, fertility is important to many women who undergo this surgery. Losing the ability to have children isn't easy and may generate a flood of emotions.

For others, entering menopause or no longer having periods, may make them feel empty or less feminine. Please know that this is not true.

If you're dealing with post-surgical grief, it's natural and okay. A hysterectomy is life-altering, and we all handle it differently. By prioritizing your mental and emotional health, you'll make it through this.

MANAGING YOUR MIND

Our thought patterns form over time. Just as you can train your body for a marathon, you can train your mind, too.

Here are a few techniques to do just that.

OBSERVE YOUR THOUGHTS.

Your thoughts aren't as random as you may believe. There's a strong link between your thoughts and past experiences, observations and biases.

Start by observing your thoughts or paying *close attention* to them. This practice can shift your perspective and how you react in various situations. It gives you the power to challenge the validity of your thoughts, manage negative thinking and improve your mental state. Here's a simple way to become more mindful of your feelings:

- Sit in a calm environment.

- Close your eyes and take a few deep breaths.

- Focus on just one thought. Determine how it came to be.

- Evaluate if your thought is based on facts and how it impacts your self-identity and well-being.

- Remind yourself that the thoughts don't control you. You control them.

WATCH THE NEGATIVE INNER CRITIC.

Did you know that 88% of us criticize ourselves in ways we would never criticize others?[55] As women, we can be highly self-critical.

To improve your mental health, break this cycle. **Identify** what your inner self is telling you, then consciously **decide to ignore** the negative self-talk. Become your own cheerleader.

Any time your inside voice says, "You are not attractive anymore" or "You're less of a woman because...," remind yourself of the challenges you've overcome.

Counter the negative thoughts with positive affirmations. Write them on post-it notes and place them around your room as a constant reminder to be kinder to yourself.

REFRAME UNHELPFUL THOUGHTS.

Once you've identified the negative self-talk, it's time to replace it with positive thoughts. **Easier said than done, I know.**

Start with changing just one unhelpful belief rather than trying to tackle everything right away. Your new way of thinking will eventually become habitual. Once you've reframed the first habit, proceed to the next one.

Over time, your mental well-being will improve.

AVOID OVERTHINKING.

Most of us are guilty of overthinking or imagining worst-case scenarios. This thought process is unhealthy and often causes anxiety or depression.

Here are a few ways to control overthinking:[56]

- Acknowledge your thoughts. Evaluate if they need as much mental energy. Reframe your approach or look at the issue from a different angle.

- Write down your thoughts and come back to them later. It'll give you time to disassociate your feelings from rational thoughts.

- Be thankful for the small milestones in your recovery. Gratitude has a way of pushing away negative feelings before they get out of control.

MANAGING YOUR EMOTIONS

A hysterectomy can exacerbate fear, anger and anxiety, causing our body's fight-or-flight response to kick in.

Managing these emotions isn't easy, but here are some tips that can help.

SEE EMOTIONS AS MESSENGERS, NOT FACTS.

Emotions are signals from our bodies and a reaction to external or internal stressors. They tell us what we're going through at a given time. If you're feeling unattractive or less feminine, understand that it's your body's reaction to your *current* state.

Try changing the incorrect signals to manage your emotions. Get a new hairdo, change your clothes, sit with your girlfriends, or do things that make you feel like yourself again.

Emotions are temporary. Try to recall past experiences where emotions felt like facts at the moment but changed over time.

LOOK FOR THE NEED BEHIND THE EMOTION.

Figure out what your feelings are trying to tell you. Think of your feelings as a person asking you to take action. Once you understand what the emotion wants you to do, you'll be in a much better place to manage it.

For example, if you're feeling overwhelmed or uneasy, perhaps you can use some alone time to reset and recognize the changes in your body. You can also journal how you're feeling, which can help you feel better.

ASKING FOR HELP

Being self-reliant is often promoted in our culture, so asking for help may seem weak. When it comes to getting advice and much-needed support, requesting help is just the opposite; it's a wise and courageous move.

Identify people you can turn to for specific tasks. These may be people in your support system (trusted family and friends) or those with special skills and knowledge, such as a counselor.

Getting help can lift a huge weight off your shoulders as you work through health and emotional challenges.

GET SUPPORT. DON'T ISOLATE.

Join online or in-person support groups for women who've had a hysterectomy. It'll give you an outlet to discuss issues others may not relate to. You'll also find resources to manage your physical and mental health.

SUPPORTIVE LIFESTYLE CHANGES

Your environment and habits can impact your mindset. Let's examine how changing your lifestyle can positively influence your mental well-being.

EXERCISE FOR A BETTER MOOD.

Exercise releases "happy" hormones (serotonin and dopamine), which fight depression, negative thinking and anxiety and improve our mood and physical health. So, engage in some movement every day.

There are no rules about how much exercise you need or which type, so do whatever makes you feel good and at a level that's safe for you.

I used to take walks in the early days after my procedure, then added strength training once my doctor approved. Exercise improved my mood and self-image, and I soon felt like myself again.

EAT HEALTHIER FOR A BETTER MOOD.

The connection between food, nutrition and mental health is stronger than many realize. Staying hydrated improves our mental health as well. Eating moderate quantities of foods like dark chocolate, berries, oats, fatty fish and coffee is good for the mind.

Food like eggs, cheese and pineapples have chemicals that boost serotonin and stabilize mood. Over-processed and sugary foods and drinks make you feel good temporarily, but they contribute to depression, anxiety and fatigue.

SLEEP BETTER FOR A BETTER MOOD.

> *"Good sleep quality plays a crucial role in maintaining positive well-being and mental health. By contrast, sleep disturbances and related daytime dysfunction are a risk factor for reporting poor mental health."*[57]
>
> *VARMA ET AL., 2021*

Sleep deprivation may lead to anger, frustration, irritability and sadness. To practice good sleep hygiene:

- Create a comfy bed.
- Ensure low lighting a few hours before bedtime.
- Maintain a consistent sleep schedule.
- Use earplugs and an eye mask if needed.

Sleep stabilizes your mood by regulating hormones and giving your body time to heal.

POSITIVE AFFIRMATIONS.

Have you ever told yourself you're having a bad day? Did you notice how much worse things seemed to get, even though they weren't as bad before? Positive affirmations work the same way, but for the better.

Repeating a positive mantra when you're feeling down removes negative thoughts from your mind. It lifts the spirit and boosts your immune system.

SOCIALIZE.

You may not feel like socializing after a hysterectomy, but the company can do you good. The COVID lockdown era is an example of how social isolation affects the mind. So, instead of isolating yourself, spend time with others and keep reasonably busy.

Invite friends and family to take your mind off the recovery. If you can't meet in person, try catching up by text or on a video call.

PRAY.

Spending time with God can change your outlook on life and release stressors beyond your control. If you're distraught, prayer can ground you, reduce tension and help you through the tough times, especially when you're dealing with loss, pain or depression.

JOURNAL.

Journaling is a powerful tool for managing your mindset before and after surgery. Writing down your thoughts can help you identify problematic patterns and analyze your feelings without judgment.

When you're having a hard day, simply revisit your journal for inspiration or to see how far you've come. You can journal your way.

I found journaling so beneficial as I worked to get my weight under control that I created my own. You can get a copy at www.hysterectomyfitness.com/journals.

WORK ON AN ATTITUDE OF GRATITUDE.

Gratitude puts things into perspective. It shifts your focus from what you lost to what you gained or retained. It also helps you stay optimistic and appreciate your blessings. To practice gratitude:

- Give thanks for *individual* things.

- Be specific. Name people and exactly what you are grateful for.

- Appreciate the little things around you.

- Vocalize your feelings. For example, if a friend helped you put the groceries away, let them know how thankful you are.

- Find a new reason to be grateful every day.

- Start and end your day with an attitude of gratitude.

Changing your thought process isn't easy. When you face setbacks or catch yourself reverting to old habits, return to these steps. I've also included a roadmap for starting your own gratitude journal at the end of this chapter.

The tips I've shared helped me improve my mindset over time. I hope you find them useful, too.

To wrap up, let's review the highlights of the chapter:

- Identify your core beliefs about a hysterectomy.

- Manage your mindset by observing your thoughts, limiting your inner critic, reframing unhelpful thoughts and avoiding overthinking.

- See your emotions as messengers, not facts of life.

- Seek help from your support system.

- Join online or in-person support groups.

- Make changes in your physical activity, nutrition and sleep to support your mood.

- Some ways to improve your mental well-being include positive affirmations, socializing, praying, journaling and practicing gratitude.

You're now caught up on *everything* you need to know about what to expect before, during and after a hysterectomy.

I know the process can be overwhelming, so I'd like to share some inspiring stories from other hysterectomy survivors. Take heart; there is a light at the end of the tunnel.

Your Roadmap to
Starting a Gratitude Journal

- ☐ Identify something good from today. It doesn't matter if it's big or small.

- ☐ Identify how you felt about it. Now, jot it down.

- ☐ Rinse and repeat.

- ☐ Write at least three things every day.

Tips to Remember:

- Include little details and expand on each point.

- Be specific.

- Remember to count the bad things that didn't happen.

- Try to include new perspectives each day instead of repeating the same thing every day.

- Don't skip. This practice is even more beneficial on bad days.

Chapter 10

REAL-LIFE STORIES OF POST-HYSTERECTOMY SURVIVORS

"Hope is being able to see that there is light despite all of the darkness."

DESMOND TUTU

Y ou may be having a difficult time right now. I hope you'll find strength knowing that others have had a hysterectomy and are now enjoying fulfilled lives. This is a testament that you can, too.

Let me introduce you to five women who had a hysterectomy for various reasons and are doing well.

52-YEAR-OLD WITH HEAVY MENSTRUAL BLEEDING

Meet Kathleen Morrissey. She's a mom and a cycling enthusiast. She suffered from heavy menstrual bleeding and had a large polyp in her uterine lining, making her give up cycling.

She underwent an endometrial ablation to fix her gynecological issues. Its success was short-lived, so she had a laparoscopic hysterectomy at 52. She had her uterus and cervix removed, but kept her ovaries.

Due to the minimally invasive surgical approach, Kathleen was home by 5 p.m. the day of surgery and back on her feet two days later. She returned to work a week and a half after her procedure.

After a few weeks, she resumed her favorite activity — long bike rides. She shares that her quality of life has significantly improved since the procedure. Her only regret is not getting a hysterectomy sooner.[58]

NAVY VETERAN WHO DEALT WITH FIBROID PAIN FOR 17 YEARS

Meet Lakisha Watson-Moore. She's a mom, an athlete and a Navy veteran who suffered from heavy menstrual bleeding due to multiple uterine fibroids.

Although she had an active lifestyle and was a regular at the gym, she struggled to maintain her weight. Lakisha went to her gynecologist at age 40 to schedule a hysterectomy when the pain became unbearable. She had an open abdominal hysterectomy because of the number of fibroids and their size.

The first few weeks of recovery were rough. Lakisha couldn't exercise. She lost muscle and had pain at her incision site. She also experienced bloating, moodiness and body temperature changes due to hormonal imbalance.

It took her several months to feel healthy again. But she is now better than ever and says that having a hysterectomy was the best decision ever.

Since the procedure, her workout quality has improved, and she can do core exercises without pain, which was impossible before. She's back to her active lifestyle and running Spartan races without excruciating pain.[59]

40-YEAR-OLD WITH ENDOMETRIOSIS

Meet Amy Schumer. She's an actress, a comedian, mom and hysterectomy survivor. She had 30 endometriosis spots in her abdomen and pelvis, which caused her unbearable pain and fertility issues.

She decided to have a hysterectomy at 40 and had her uterus and appendix removed.

She's been on a fitness journey since the procedure and feels "like a new person". She's most happy about not being in debilitating pain for most of the month. It's given her freedom and lifted the mental exhaustion that came with the pain.[60]

FERTILITY ISSUES, MISCARRIAGE AND ANEMIA

Meet Viola Davis. She's an actress and a producer. She had uterine fibroids, fertility issues and heavy bleeding for years, which made her extremely anemic.

In her early 30's, she had surgery to remove her uterine fibroids. When that didn't work, she had a myomectomy to remove over 30 fibroids. Then, a few years later, she had a hysterectomy that removed her uterus and fallopian tubes.

Since the procedure, she has mentioned struggles with weight management. But she's been doing well overall. Not having periods has freed her from being in constant pain and bleeding.

She actively works out and trains professionally for challenging roles.[61]

WOMAN IN HER 40S WITH COUNTLESS FIBROIDS

Meet Melanie Durette. She is a fitness enthusiast and personal coach. She had uterine fibroids and suffered from heavy and prolonged bleeding for nearly a decade.

She mostly wore black clothes and loose shirts because she feared bleeding through her pad. Her wardrobe made her feel less feminine. The excessive bleeding also made it difficult to train consistently.

Melanie decided to have a total laparoscopic hysterectomy when she couldn't live the life she wanted because she lacked energy.

She calls the procedure "a gift to myself" because it gave her her life back. Melanie's most significant upsides from the surgery are:

- She can wear colored clothes again.
- She can train as much as she wants because her energy levels are good.
- She doesn't have to plan her life around periods that knocked her out for 2-3 weeks.

Melanie proactively trains her pelvic floor to prevent prolapse. She's also managed to maintain her weight and fitness with diet and exercise.[62]

Several other women have turned their lives around after having a hysterectomy. By using the knowledge in this book, you too can position yourself for success after surgery and get your life back.

Thank you!

Thank you for your purchase! If you've enjoyed this book, please let me know how it's helped you better prepare for surgery or come out mentally and physically stronger.

Many women are still misinformed about a hysterectomy and base their decisions on fear, myths and misconceptions. Others are struggling with post-hysterectomy symptoms and need help navigating these issues.

Please consider sharing your review on Amazon to spread the word and help more women benefit from this resource so they can be inspired, too.

To leave a review, scan the QR code below using your phone's camera or the link in your Amazon order to launch the review page.

It only takes 60 seconds.

Conclusion

"He who has health, has hope; and he who has hope, has everything."

THOMAS CARLYLE

Here are the key takeaways from each chapter.

- There are different types of hysterectomies: **Total,** with **salpingo-oophorectomy** (removal of ovaries and fallopian tubes), **supracervical** and **radical.**

- You can choose an **abdominal,** a **vaginal** or minimally invasive/**laparoscopic** surgery.

- Uterine fibroids, endometriosis and precancerous and cancerous cells in the gynecological organs are a few of the most common **reasons for having a hysterectomy.**

- You'll go into **menopause immediately if your ovaries are removed**.

- Changes in **libido and orgasm** depend on the type of hysterectomy and psychological factors.

- Hysterectomy is the last resort for issues with the female reproductive system, not the go-to choice.

- There won't just be a space inside you after a hysterectomy. The remaining internal **organs will shift into place. Recovery time depends on the type** of hysterectomy, with minimally invasive surgery having the quickest recovery. It may take you longer or shorter to heal, depending on why you had the procedure.

- To prepare for a hysterectomy, **ask questions** and understand your treatment **options.** Weigh the **pros**

and cons, but **don't delay** surgery unnecessarily.

- Quit smoking **before the procedure**. Try to include high-fiber ingredients in your diet and lose weight if you're overweight.

- The surgery takes 1-2 hours. You may return home within 24 hours or up to five days, depending on why you had the surgery. Ask your doctor if you can take your regular medications on surgery day.

- **After the procedure,** you may be nauseous, bloated and constipated and bleed for a few days. Don't soak your fresh wound. Wash your hands before tending to your wounds. Expect pain at the surgical site and your throat, back and possibly, hips and joints.

- Wait six weeks to have **penetrative sex**. Try not to carry heavy objects during this time or overdo physical activities. You may still have kids (but no pregnancy) after a hysterectomy. You may still have light periods, but contact your doctor if your bleeding increases or lasts longer than a few weeks.

- Start **prepping for the surgery two months before.** Create a support system and consult a mental health professional if you need additional support. Try to reduce stressors.

- Do these at least **a month before:** Sort out your insurance. Learn about the type of limitations you'll have following surgery. Apply for medical leave.

- Shop for necessities and fill your fridge **a week before the surgery.** Prepare quick meals and freeze them. Ready your room, finish chores and pre-fill your prescriptions.

- Try to relax your mind through deep breathing **the day before.** Prep your body with antiseptic soap and shower. Get your hospital bag ready.

- **On surgery day,** you will fill out hospital forms and move into your hospital room. You'll change into a backless gown, be wheeled to surgery and given anesthesia. After surgery, you may wake up with a sore throat. Try to walk soon afterward to alleviate constipation and blood clots.

- Your **wound heals** in phases and will fully recover in about two years. Watch out for infections while the wound is fresh.

- It's okay to sleep a lot during the **first week at home.** Eating a high-fiber diet and drinking plenty of water will alleviate constipation. Try to move regularly. Take pain medications before the pain is unbearable. Follow your doctor's guidelines for wound care and take care of your mental health.

- **Post-op complications** may include early menopause, infections, blood clots, pain, weight gain, weight management difficulties, urinary leakage, pelvic muscle weakness and organ prolapse.

- **Identity your core beliefs** about hysterectomy by observing your thoughts, limiting your inner critic, reframing unhelpful thoughts and not overthinking.

- To **manage your mindset,** seek help from your support system. Join online or in-person support groups and make healthy lifestyle changes. Socialization, prayer, journaling and practicing gratitude can regulate your emotions.

I was not a picture of health going into surgery. My recovery afterward wasn't smooth sailing either. I had tough days where I couldn't exercise or eat without gaining weight. I felt helpless on those days, and it made me miserable. But today, my health and fitness are a thousand times better than I ever imagined they could be.

The information I've shared in this book is the fusion of my knowledge and experience of post-op recovery from the past six years. I am where I am because I practiced these recovery tips.

My sincere hope is that the topics I've covered in this book will help you better prepare for your hysterectomy or come out of it mentally and physically stronger.

I wish you all the best and a full life after all the pain and suffering you've been through. You can do this!

Citations

1 NCI Dictionary of Cancer Terms. (n.d.). National Cancer Institute. https://www.cancer.gov/publications/dictionaries/cancer-terms

2 Types. (2017, September 12). Stanford Health Care. https://stanfordhealthcare.org/medical-treatments/h/hysterectomy/types.html

3 Website, N. (2023, July 24). Hysterectomy. nhs.uk. https://www.nhs.uk/conditions/hysterectomy/

4 Zaritsky, E., Ojo, A., Tucker, L., & Raine-Bennett, T. (2019). Racial disparities in route of hysterectomy for benign indications within an integrated health care system. JAMA Network Open, 2(12), e1917004. https://doi.org/10.1001/jamanetworkopen.2019.17004

5 Manning, C., Gompers, A., Hacker, & Jorgensen, E. (2022). Racial and ethnic disparities in utilization of Minimally-Invasive Hysterectomy. Journal of Minimally Invasive Gynecology, 29(11), S11–S12. https://doi.org/10.1016/j.jmig.2022.09.046

6 Bougie, O., Healey, J., & Singh, S. S. (2019). Behind the times: revisiting endometriosis and race. American Journal of Obstetrics and Gynecology, 221(1), 35.e1-35.e5. https://doi.org/10.1016/j.ajog.2019.01.238

7 Professional, C. C. M. (n.d.). Hysterectomy. Cleveland Clinic. https://my.clevelandclinic.org/health/treatments/4852-hysterectomy

8 Bossick, A. S., Sangha, R., Olden, H., Alexander, G., & Wegienka, G. (2018). Identifying what matters to hysterectomy patients: postsurgery perceptions, beliefs, and experiences. Journal of Patient-Centered Research and Reviews, 5(2), 167–175. https://doi.org/10.17294/2330-0698.1581

9 Madueke-Laveaux, O. S., Elsharoud, A., & Al-Hendy, A. (2021). What We Know about the Long-Term Risks of Hysterectomy for Benign Indication — A Systematic Review. Journal of Clinical Medicine, 10(22), 5335. https://doi.org/10.3390/jcm10225335

10 Danesh, M., Hamzehgardeshi, Z., Moosazadeh, M., & Shabani-Asrami, F. (2015). The Effect of Hysterectomy on Women's Sexual Function: a Narrative Review. Medicinski Arhiv, 69(6), 387. https://doi.org/10.5455/medarh.2015.69.387-392

11 Rhodes, J., Kjerulff, K. H., & Langenberg, P. (1999). Hysterectomy and sexual functioning. JAMA, 282(20), 1934. https://doi.org/10.1001/jama.282.20.1934

12 Ferhi, M., Abdeljabbar, A., Jaballah, F., Jihenne, M., & Nadia, M. (2023). Impact on sexual functioning: total versus subtotal hysterectomy. Research Square (Research Square). https://doi.org/10.21203/rs.3.rs-2551130/v1

13 Eunice Kennedy Shriver National Institute of Child Health and Human Development - NICHD. (n.d.). https://www.nichd.nih.gov/health/topics/factsheets/uterine

14 Professional, C. C. M. (n.d.). Hysterectomy. Cleveland Clinic. https://my.clevelandclinic.org/health/treatments/4852-hysterectomy

15 Berzins, K. (2022, May 15). The facts and myths about having a hysterectomy - McLeod Health. McLeod Health. https://www.mcleodhealth.org/blog/the-facts-and-myths-about-having-a-hysterectomy/

16 Lunde, S., Nguyen, H. T., Petersen, K. K., Arendt-Nielsen, L., Krarup, H., & Søgaard-Andersen, E. (2020). Chronic postoperative pain after hysterectomy for endometrial cancer: A Metabolic Profiling study. Molecular Pain, 16, 174480692092388. https://doi.org/10.1177/1744806920923885

17 Website, N. (2022, October 14). Complications. nhs.uk. https://www.nhs.uk/conditions/hysterectomy/risks

18 Moorman, P. G., Myers, E. R., Schildkraut, J. M., Iversen, E. S., Wang, F., & Warren, N. (2011). Effect of hysterectomy with ovarian

preservation on ovarian function. Obstetrics & Gynecology, 118(6), 1271–1279. https://doi.org/10.1097/aog.0b013e318236fd12

19 Madueke-Laveaux, O. S., Elsharoud, A., & Al-Hendy, A. (2021). What We Know about the Long-Term Risks of Hysterectomy for Benign Indication — A Systematic Review. Journal of Clinical Medicine, 10(22), 5335. https://doi.org/10.3390/jcm10225335

20 Post hysterectomy vaginal vault prolapse | Tampa General. (n.d.). https://www.tgh.org/institutes-and-services/conditions/post-hysterectomy-vaginal-vault-prolapse

21 Li, P. C., Tsai, I., Hsu, C. Y., Wang, J. H., Lin, S., Ding, D., & Sung, F. C. (2018). Risk of Hyperlipidemia in Women with Hysterectomy-A Retrospective Cohort Study in Taiwan. Scientific Reports, 8(1). https://doi.org/10.1038/s41598-018-31347-z

22 Hysterectomy associated with an increased risk of cardiovascular disease, study says - Mayo Clinic. (2020b, April 23). https://www.mayoclinic.org/medical-professionals/obstetrics-gynecology/news/hysterectomy-associated-with-an-increased-risk-of-cardiovascular-disease-study-says/mac-20476157

23 Alkatout, İ., Mettler, L., Peters, G., Noé, G. K., Holthaus, B., Jonat, W., & Schollmeyer, T. (2014). Laparoscopic Hysterectomy and Prolapse: a multiprocedural concept. JSLS, 18(1), 89–101. https://doi.org/10.4293/108680813x13693422520846

24 Bakalar, N. (2019, October 1). Hysterectomy may raise depression and anxiety risk. The New York Times. https://www.nytimes.com/2019/10/01/well/mind/hysterectomy-may-raise-depression-and-anxiety-risk.html

25 Fletcher, J. (2023, March 31). Hysterectomy side effects and recovery. https://www.medicalnewstoday.com/articles/hysterectomy-side-effects

26 Website, N. (2022b, October 14). Complications. nhs.uk. https://www.nhs.uk/conditions/hysterectomy/risks/

27 ABC News. (2015, March 25). Angelina Jolie's surgery and what you should know. ABC News. https://abcnews.go.com/Health/angelina-jolies-surgery/story?id=29865394

28 Website, N. (2021, November 18). Can I eat or drink before an operation? nhs.uk. https://www.nhs.uk/common-health-questions/operations-tests-and-procedures/can-i-eat-or-drink-before-an-operation/

29 Gordon, B. S. (2012, May 11). Is combining hysterectomy and a tummy tuck safe? Medical Xpress. https://medicalxpress.com/news/2012-05-combining-hysterectomy-tummy-tuck-safe.html

30 Total & surpacervical hysterectomy (Partial hysterectomy) | CU OB-GYN. (2019, April 4). University of Colorado OB-GYN. https://obgyn.coloradowomenshealth.com/services/surgeries/hysterectomy/partial-hysterectomy

31 Modesty during hysterectomy. (n.d.). http://patientmodesty.org/hysterectomymodesty.aspx

32 Tarigonda, S., Manem, A., Shenoy, K. U., Duggappa, A. K. H., & Krishna, R. (2021). Comparison of intravenous ondansetron, ramosetron and palonosetron for prevention of postoperative nausea and vomiting in patients undergoing total abdominal hysterectomy: a RCT. Journal of Clinical and Diagnostic Research. https://doi.org/10.7860/jcdr/2021/50592.15655

33 Krafft, N. (2022, June 9). Is bloating after surgery normal? Nutrisense Journal. https://www.nutrisense.io/blog/is-bloating-after-surgery-normal

34 Bleeding after a hysterectomy | Sutter Health. (n.d.). https://www.sutterhealth.org/ask-an-expert/answers/bleeding-after-a-hysterectomy

35 Lyngdoh, B., Kriplani, A., Garg, P., Maheshwari, D., & Bansal, R. (2009). Post-hysterectomy menstruation: a rare phenomenon. Archives of Gynecology and Obstetrics, 281(2), 307–309. https://doi.org/10.1007/s00404-009-1173-2

36 Fylstra, D. L. (2015). Ectopic pregnancy after hysterectomy may not be so uncommon: A case report and review of the literature. Case Reports in Women's Health, 7, 8–11. https://doi.org/10.1016/j.crwh.2015.04.001

37 Clarke-Pearson, D. L., & Geller, E. J. (2013). Complications of hysterectomy. Obstetrics & Gynecology, 121(3), 654–673. https://doi.org/10.1097/aog.0b013e3182841594

38 Techniques. (2017, September 12). Stanford Health Care. https://stanfordhealthcare.org/medical-treatments/h/hysterectomy/techniques.html

39 Hysterectomy. (n.d.). Mount Sinai Health System. https://www.mountsinai.org/health-library/surgery/hysterectomy

40 Hysterectomy Patient success Story | Beaumont Health. (n.d.). https://www.beaumont.org/services/womens-services/gynecology-services/gynecologic-surgery/hysterectomy-patient-success-story

41 Video: Amy Schumer in hospital as she undergoes endometriosis surgery | Daily Mail Online. (n.d.). Mail Online. http://www.dailymail.co.uk/video/tvshowbiz/video-2505769/Video-Amy-Schumer-hospital-undergoes-endometriosis-surgery.html

42 Diane. (2023, February 28). Hysterectomy – Talia's Story - Cherokee Women's Health. Cherokee Women's Health. https://cherokeewomenshealth.com/2019/07/hysterectomy-talias-story/

43 Cws, S. D. M. R. (2021, February 22). How long does it take a surgical incision to heal? | Sanara MedTech. Sanara MedTech. https://sanaramedtech.com/blog/how-long-for-surgical-incision-to-heal/

44 [Feeling of illness after hysterectomy. Women's own assessment]. (2001, December 10). PubMed. https://pubmed.ncbi.nlm.nih.gov/11794034/

45 UpToDate. (n.d.). UpToDate. https://www.uptodate.com/contents/care-after-gynecologic-surgery-beyond-the-basics/

46 Lin, Y. H., & Li, T. S. (2016). The application of Far-Infrared in the treatment of wound healing. Journal of Evidence-Based Complementary & Alternative Medicine, 22(1), 186–188. https://doi.org/10.1177/2156587215623436

47 Madueke-Laveaux, O. S., Elsharoud, A., & Al-Hendy, A. (2021b). What We Know about the Long-Term Risks of Hysterectomy

for Benign Indication — A Systematic Review. Journal of Clinical Medicine, 10(22), 5335. https://doi.org/10.3390/jcm10225335

48 Chan, C. X., & Nimaroff, M. (2022). Surgical Site Infection after Hysterectomy. In IntechOpen eBooks. https://doi.org/10.5772/intechopen.101492

49 Clarke-Pearson, D. L., & Geller, E. J. (2013b). Complications of hysterectomy. Obstetrics & Gynecology, 121(3), 654–673. https://doi.org/10.1097/aog.0b013e3182841594

50 Knight, M. G., Anekwe, C. V., Krystilyn, W., Akam, E. Y., Wang, E., & Stanford, F. C. (2021). Weight regulation in menopause. Menopause, 28(8), 960–965. https://doi.org/10.1097/gme.0000000000001792

51 Chen, V., Shackelford, L., & Spain, M. (2021). Pelvic floor dysfunction after hysterectomy: Moving the investigation forward. Cureus. https://doi.org/10.7759/cureus.15661

52 Post hysterectomy vaginal vault prolapse | Tampa General. (n.d.-b). https://www.tgh.org/institutes-and-services/conditions/post-hysterectomy-vaginal-vault-prolapse

53 Dällenbach, P., Kaelin-Gambirasio, I., Dubuisson, J., & Boulvain, M. (2007). Risk factors for pelvic organ prolapse repair after hysterectomy. Obstetrics & Gynecology, 110(3), 625–632. https://doi.org/10.1097/01.aog.0000278567.37925.4e

54 Gabriel, I., Kalousdian, A., Brito, L. G. O., Abdalian, T., Vitonis, A. F., & Minassian, V. A. (2021). Pelvic organ prolapse after 3 modes of hysterectomy: long-term follow-up. American Journal of Obstetrics and Gynecology, 224(5), 496.e1-496.e10. https://doi.org/10.1016/j.ajog.2020.11.008

55 Mortimer, C. (2016, January 4). Women criticise themselves an average of eight times a day, study says | The Independent. The Independent. https://www.independent.co.uk/life-style/health-and-families/health-news/women-criticise-themselves-an-average-of-eight-times-a-day-study-says-a6796286.html

56 Maenpaa, J. (2022, February 25). A psychotherapist shares the 3 exercises she uses every day "to stop overthinking." CNBC. https://www.cnbc.com/2022/02/25/a-psychotherapist-shares-the-exercises-she-uses-every-day-to-stop-overthinking.html

57 Varma, P., Burge, M., Meaklim, H., Junge, M., & Jackson, M. L. (2021). Poor Sleep Quality and Its Relationship with Individual Characteristics, Personal Experiences and Mental Health during the COVID-19 Pandemic. International Journal of Environmental Research and Public Health, 18(11), 6030. https://doi.org/10.3390/ijerph18116030

58 Robotic Hysterectomy patient Story. (n.d.). (C)1998-2023 Geonetric. All Rights Reserved. https://www.milfordregional.org/social-media/patient-stories/gynecology/robotic-laparoscopic-hysterectomy/

59 Watson-Moore, L. (2020, August 12). After my hysterectomy, I'm living my best life. HealthyWomen. https://www.healthywomen.org/real-women-real-stories/after-my-hysterectomy-im-living-my-best-life

60 Walsh, K. (2022, December 13). Amy Schumer Opens Up About Hysterectomy to Treat Endometriosis. Glamour. https://www.glamour.com/story/amy-schumer-talks-endometriosis-life-changing-magic-of-a-hysterectomy

61 Yahoo is part of the Yahoo family of brands. (n.d.). https://www.yahoo.com/lifestyle/viola-davis-shares-she-had-hysterectomy-reveals-she-threatened-to-kick-surgeons-ass-if-i-wake-up-and-my-uterus-is-still-here-192851576.html

62 Durette, M., & Durette, M. (2022). My Positive Hysterectomy Story – Getting My Life Back After 10 Years Of Heavy Bleeding | Female Fitness Systems. Female Fitness Systems. https://femalefitnesssystems.com/my-positive-hysterectomy-story/

My Other Books

- Hysterectomy Fitness Weight-Loss Journal for Women (Book 1): Your 12-Week Planner to Track and Maintain Weight Loss Before, During & After Surgery

- Hysterectomy Fitness Weight-Loss Journal for Women (Book 2): Your 12-Week Planner and Mind-Body Roadmap to Lose Weight and Boost Metabolism After Surgery

Printed in Great Britain
by Amazon

60789262R00107